Rehabilitation
of Stroke

Rehabilitation of Stroke

Paul E. Kaplan, M.D.
Medical Director
Rehabilitation Management Systems
Sacramento, California
Honorary Professor
University of British Columbia Faculty of Medicine
Vancouver, Canada

Rene Cailliet, M.D.
Clinical Professor
Department of Rehabilitation Medicine
University of Southern California School of Medicine
Los Angeles, California

Candia P. Kaplan, Ph.D., A.B.P.P.
Manager, Health Psychology and Internship Training Director
Psychiatric Services
Ball Memorial Hospital
Muncie, Indiana

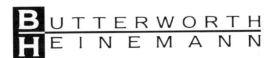

BUTTERWORTH
HEINEMANN

An Imprint of Elsevier Science

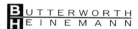
An imprint of Elsevier Science

200 Wheeler Road
Burlington, MA 01803

Rehabilitation of Stroke   0-7506-7432-6

Notice

Physical medicine and rehabilitation is an ever-changing field. Standard safety precautions must be followed, but as new research and clinical experience broaden our knowledge, changes in treatment and drug therapy may become necessary or appropriate. Readers are advised to check the most current product information provided by the manufacturer of each drug to be administered to verify the recommended dose, the method and duration of administration, and contraindications. It is the responsibility of the treating physician, relying on experience and knowledge of the patient, to determine dosages and the best treatment for each individual patient. Neither the Publisher nor the author assume any liability for any injury and/or damage to persons or property arising from this publication.

The Publisher

Library of Congress Cataloging-in-Publication Data
Kaplan, Paul E., 1940-
   Rehabilitation of stroke / Paul E. Kaplan, Rene Cailliet, Candia P. Kaplan.—1st ed.
    p. cm.
   ISBN 0-7506-7432-6
   1. Cerebrovascular disease—Patients—Rehabilitation. I. Cailliet, Rene. II. Kaplan, Candia P. III. Title.

RC388.5 .K364 2003
616.8'103—dc21

          2002026153

Executive Publisher: Kim Murphy
Editorial Assistant: Meghan McGlone
Project Manager: Mary Stermel

SSC/MVY

Printed in the United States of America.

Last digit is the print number: 9 8 7 6 5 4 3 2 1

4/14/03

Contents

C. TREATMENT OF OUTPATIENTS

Preface

Currently in the United States, two out of every three people will be significantly disabled before they die. As our population ages, many of these disabled people will have incurred a stroke syndrome, will experience weakness, and will be dependent. They will not be able to be self-sufficient in their home communities.

Stroke syndromes are not a homogenous group. They are varied in causation and presentation, but all are characterized by vascular supply failure to portions of the central nervous system. Before treatment or rehabilitation, the treating physician will recognize specific clinical patterns and specific resultant functional impairment.

This text focuses on the evaluation of patients who have had hemorrhagic strokes as a basis for determining management strategies vital to rehabilitation of patients with stroke disorders. The fact that patients with hemorrhagic strokes have maximal functional capacities in their adult years and also usually possess enormous potential for anatomic, physiologic, and functional return means that the rehabilitation medicine process could achieve spectacular results—self-sufficient patients able to return to their home communities. To generate this type of optimal outcome, the full clinical group of professionals disciplined in different medical areas needs to understand the nature and role of each of the components of the patient's overall clinical neurofunctional rehabilitation potential and to act effectively as one unified, spirited team to achieve that patient's maximal clinical neurofunctional recovery.

There are many premorbid factors that influence neurologic function, such as obesity, poor lifestyle habits, and significant physiologic diseases such as hypertension and diabetes. These factors can limit a patient's neurofunctional recovery and must be managed. However, once the stroke has been manifested, these premorbid factors could be thought of as merely adjunct conditions. With hemorrhagic stroke disorders, if preventive measures are not undertaken in time, the original stroke disorder could promptly return.

The primary treating physician, who usually is the initial evaluator and manager, performs the accepted, standard neurologic testing. However, this standard neurologic testing is often not fully adequate for that physician to understand how these particular neurologic findings have led to the patient's specific impairment. With inadequate understanding of neurologic impairment, an appropriate curative or managerial treatment protocol cannot be applied. Specialized radiologic scans are no substitute for an effective, efficient neurologic evaluation. Optimal functional advances will not be realized without a thorough, accurate, clinical neurologic evaluation. This text is intended to answer challenges posed by stroke disorders in the context of a clinical neurologic evaluation.

The clinical neurologic pattern, the curative and managerial treatment, and the rehabilitative care of hemorrhagic stroke are different than for thrombotic stroke. The results of the clinical neurologic functional evaluation will differ between the types of stroke as will the resulting treatment protocol. The age of the patient, the amount of progressive heart disease, and the potential for stroke return or for recovery from stroke also differ between thrombotic and hemorrhagic strokes. The team approach that is advocated will also not be the same as the stroke evolves through differing clinical stages. All of the team efforts influence the ultimate functional prognosis for stroke patients. The common factor is the application of the functional neurologic clinical examination, which leads to a more meaningful treatment and also a better prognosis.

Therapeutic rehabilitative prescription rests squarely on the clinical application of examination results to the creation of a rehabilitation contract between the patient, the rehabilitation case manager, and the rest of the rehabilitation team. However, physicians' authority rests, in part, on their ability to bring to the team the context and interpretation of the patient's clinical neurologic functional examination findings. These physicians' leadership and facilitative abilities to lead the team in rehabilitative treatment depend on the implications of their neurologic functional evaluations.

As the clinical course of the stroke unfolds after the hemorrhage, the management setting usually evolves from acute inpatient care to outpatient follow-up treatment. During the transition, the membership of the rehabilitation team also changes in number, discipline, and personnel as the environmental characteristics of rehabilitation change. Therefore, although the fundamental contract of rehabilitative treatment also changes, progress and momentum toward independence of the patient should continue. This book presents a road map through the trials and tribulations of rehabilitative care of stroke patients aimed at the ultimate success of the rehabilitation medicine process.

Paul E. Kaplan, M.D.

A

Clinical Presentation

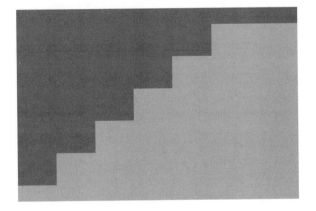

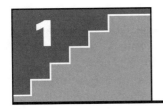

Parietal Lobe Hand

Paul E. Kaplan

More than 60% of hospitalized patients with cerebrovascular disease survive, but over 70% of those who do survive are disabled.[1,2] Almost 5% require total care. Stroke might be a bit more frequent in men than women, but this finding has been controversial.[3–6] Death rates are influenced by age, which affects men and women equally.[7] Since the 1970s, medications have been created to manage hyperlipidemia, hypertension, myocardial infarctions, and heart failure. Intensive care monitoring of patients with acute coronary artery disease has accompanied cardiac catheter laboratory procedures, angioplasty, and even cardiothoracic surgical procedures such as cardiac and pulmonary transplantation. Survival after thrombotic stroke in particular has been limited by progressive heart disease. Although reductions have therefore been made in death rates studied during the initial 30 days after stroke, the overall incidence of stroke remains remarkably even. Improvements in control of hypertension have been coupled with the appearance of stroke after cardiothoracic surgical and coronary artery invasive procedures. Stroke as a disabling disease will be with us for some time to come.

Rehabilitation of the patient with a hemorrhagic stroke disorder starts with the determination of the rehabilitation potential. Rehabilitation potential in turn is generated through the accurate, thorough study of that patient's neurologic clinical functional status. This section elaborates on that status. Relevant information about posture, sensation, strength, coordination, and reflexes generated by specific neuropathologic lesions are described. The goal is to facilitate efforts to compare and contrast different clinical neurologic findings to influence and guide the evolution of the full rehabilitation effort.

POSTURE OF THE UPPER LIMB

Diagrams dating back to the old kingdom in Egypt demonstrate that the posture of the parietally deficient upper limb has been observed for thousands of years. Many of these presentations are based on stretch reflexes, with both monosynaptic and polysynaptic latencies integrated at the spinal cord or medulla[8] Other reflexes contributing to posture are supportive, or righting, reflexes and tonic neck reflexes. These are routinely coordinated through the brain stem and cerebellum. Deficits in cerebral neurophysiologic function are translated into specific motor postures literally freezing these reflexes in place. This same result can take place in normal people undergoing extreme physical effort and stress.[9] In these cases, the effect of those stresses is so great that thinking people are changed to primitive, primordial status. The parietal lobe upper limb posture is as follows:

1. Attitude: flexed
2. Shoulder adducted and held in forward flexion
3. Elbow flexed and supinated
4. Wrist flexed
5. Thumb adducted
6. Fingers clenched over the thumb

Once the period of shock has ended, the antigravity musculature of the parietal upper limb has assumed the position of least stretch. Each muscle contracts and can become obstructed by fibrosis.

Should the period of shock and flaccid paralysis after a stroke be prolonged, residual downward subluxation of the humeral head—the "sloppy shoulder"—is observed. This subluxation is driven by gravity, as the state of friction between intact cartilaginous surfaces holding the shoulder joint in place is less than that between blocks of ice, and the distracting weight of the upper limb generating the subluxation is commonly in excess of 15 lb.[10–25] Even when shock and flaccid paralysis ends and spasticity begins, glenohumeral subluxation is usually fixed and maintained. Brachial plexus injury in the upper trunk can be superimposed on this evolution. As shock is replaced by spasticity after brachial plexitis, the basic upper limb posture is still maintained. Nonetheless, examination often reveals that the proximal muscles of the upper trunk distribution have become weak and have remained flaccid.

The upper limb with deficient input from the parietal lobe does not have palmar abduction of the thumb nor precise, coordinated placement of the hand in space. What movement remains to the parietal upper limb is usually patterned—a flexor synergy. Additionally, the parietal lobe hand cannot be voluntarily, consistently placed at any one specific point in space. Functional grasp capacity is greatly reduced. The seeming permanence of this posture commonly generates depression in the rehabilitation team trying to restore upper limb function.

SENSATION OF THE UPPER LIMB

Sensation can be thought of as providing completely meaningful biofeedback information but, in reality, not all sensation provides vital, strategic feedback data that can be applied toward planning future motor action sequences. Some sensation can provide distraction from specific clinical functional goals rather than aid. Recently, in a medical self assessment case report on chronic pain syndrome, during the physical examination of the patient, the sensation was summarized as the findings after pin prick, light touch, and vibration stimulation. All three of these stimulations are really static, along with heat, cold, and position, and not nearly as important to determining or planning subsequent upper limb clinical function as is dynamic sensation. Dynamic sensation does provide strategically vital information that can be used to plan motor action sequences useful for performing functional tasks. Dynamic sensation measurements are obtained through moving the examining instrument used through space (Figure 1.1).

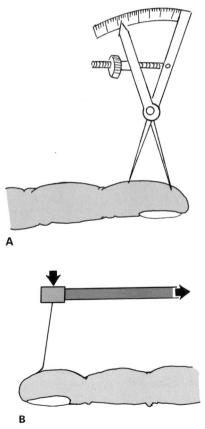

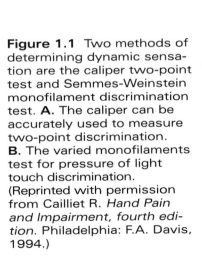

Figure 1.1 Two methods of determining dynamic sensation are the caliper two-point test and Semmes-Weinstein monofilament discrimination test. **A.** The caliper can be accurately used to measure two-point discrimination. **B.** The varied monofilaments test for pressure of light touch discrimination. (Reprinted with permission from Cailliet R. *Hand Pain and Impairment, fourth edition.* Philadelphia: F.A. Davis, 1994.)

Dynamic sensation is evaluated during the examination of two-point discrimination, stereognosis, or relative velocity determination. With these sensations, the extremity of the limb needs to be able to report motion as it moves through space.[10-20] Dynamic sensation is affected earlier, more completely, and recovers more slowly than static sensation. Of the three tests, two-point discrimination is the least sensitive but the one part of dynamic sensation testing often performed because it is relatively easy to quantify. The procedure for the two-point discrimination evaluation is as follows:

1. Metal engineering calipers are required. Use the pointed measuring ends.
2. The two points should be applied simultaneously.
3. Each observer should have experience measuring several hundred patients with normal sensation to obtain normative data pertaining to the way he or she obtains measurements.

Results of studying dynamic sensation can help clarify the clinical presentation pattern of the stroke patient. Anything that blocks or interferes with the intact sensory axis from the cerebral hemispheres—the cerebrospinal tract to the peripheral nerve—affects this evaluation. Twenty-five percent of the time, dynamic sensation is absent after a person has had a hemorrhagic stroke, even when static sensation is completely intact.[11-21] It is both tactically and strategically vital. Without dynamic sensation, a patient is not able to accurately judge how that limb is moving through space. It is vital for dressing, grooming, gait, transfer, and homemaking activities. Stereognosis is, however, more sensitive and responsive than two-point discrimination. The procedure for evaluating stereognosis is as follows:

1. A blunt stick with a relatively narrow end (a chop stick) is required.
2. Tell the patient to close his or her eyes and that you will use the stick to write one of three numbers on his or her skin. Use the same phrases each time word for word.
3. Write two, then four, then eight on the patient's forehead. After each figure is drawn, tell the patient this is how to draw a ____, and you want him or her to guess what number is drawn. Tell him or her he or she will not be penalized for guessing.
4. When the patient has been successfully instructed in the procedure, test the limb. It is recommended that you first slowly draw each figure on a proximal portion of the limb to be tested so the patient

becomes used to the evaluation. Then test the part of the limb in question using an improved technique.

5.   Hesitation or changing an answer should be counted as a deficit result, even if the response itself is correct.

The test does not take a long time. It is sensitive and specific to parietal lobe dysfunction, particularly if the soles of the feet as well as the palms of the hands are examined. Twenty-five percent of the time, specific dynamic sensory loss patterns are detected, even in the absence of deficits in static sensation (e.g., light touch and pin prick). Once a test of dynamic sensation has been performed, it usually remains a strategic part of the physical examination.

One characteristic of the musculoskeletal system is the presence of biofeedback loops. These loops are neuronal pathways that incorporate a response back to original initiating neurons as a major part of the overall neuronal outflow. For example, each smaller group of alpha motor neuron axons that exits from the anterior spine segment has axons with branches that return back to the original initiating group of alpha motor neurons. The object is to modify the activity of the original group of neurons even as those neurons change the activity of other neurons. These biofeedback loops are particularly important in providing fine-tuned motor coordination and muscular response as they increase the overall neuronal activity and provide more grades and types of positive, or activating, and negative, or inhibitory, influences within the central nervous system (Figure 1.2).

Biofeedback loops from small groups of neurons have their correlates within larger pathways of the central nervous system in reverberating neuronal pathways that link one set of nuclei to other sets.[15-19] Reverberating pathways are those pathways within the central nervous system that influence activity of other sets of neurons while also maintaining part of the pathway that modifies the activity of the originating set of neurons. The limbic lobe, for example, modifies the actions of other sets of neurons even as it changes its own activity. Reverberation enhances the function of each neuronal set in incremental stages.

Specific functional abilities are dependent on intact reverberating pathways. Both motor and sensory reverberating pathways exist. Dynamic sensation requires one such intact central nervous system sensory reverberating loop—from the parietal lobe through the frontal lobe to the lenticular nuclei to the thalamus and from the thalamus to the parietal lobe. Characteristically, dynamic sensation is obliterated at an early stage after ictus when hemorrhage and its effects have involved the anterior parietal lobe and posterior frontal lobe interrupting that pathway.[19-24]

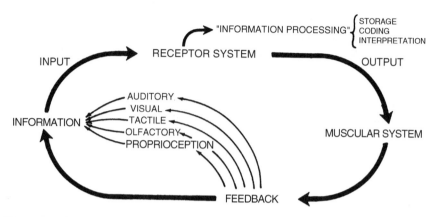

Figure 1.2 A biofeedback loop within the musculoskeletal system. Information and external environment via receptors involved in the process of learning a skill. Almost all behavior is motor in nature: Humans respond with voluntary and involuntary movements, which include posture. The learning of skills proceeds in phases. Feedback is one of the most important concepts in learning and is an important factor in the control of movement and behavior. (Reprinted with permission from Cailliet R. *Pain: Mechanisms and Management.* Philadelphia: F.A. Davis, 1993.)

Should the reverberating pathway supporting dynamic sensation be interrupted, the patient will blindly move the limb through space because he or she will not accurately receive feedback regarding its moment-to-moment position while it is in motion. In hemorrhagic strokes, dynamic sensation in the parietal lobe hand will commonly return briefly within 3 days after ictus, after the patient has been neurologically and medically stabilized, only to disappear again over the following week. Interrupting the sensory reverberating pathway as outlined in effect blinds that patient to the location of his or her limb in space. Late dynamic sensation loss frequently blocks functional return (including dressing and grooming activities) that depends on using that particular parietal lobe hand.

STRENGTH AND TONE OF THE UPPER LIMB

With time, the tone of the parietal lobe hand increases, but the strength of that hand does not increase. That increasing muscular tone—hypertonicity—does not necessarily directly evolve to classical spasticity or block motor function as spasticity does. Spasticity does modify and at times obstructs sequential motor control. For example, if spasticity is an interfering factor, the therapeutic effect of systemic medication can be augmented by the use of botulinum toxin placed periodically in strategic muscles (Figure 1.3).

What is usually observed in patients after hemorrhagic strokes is a mixture of spasticity from pyramidal involvement and rigidity from extrapyramidal involvement. This combination produces a plastic rigidity. Antigravity muscles are continuously stimulated as the tested joint continually moves through space. Cogwheel rigidity and clasp knife spasticity are both absent. Plastic rigidity is therefore formed by dysfunctional pyramidal and extrapyramidal control, but plastic rigidity itself also destroys willed isolated motor control. For example, distal muscles with plastic rigidity are recruited in an abnormal pattern when recorded using electromyography—slow firing of motor neurons even with an attempted maximal motor contraction of a joint.[20–25]

Plastic rigidity is directly associated with interruption of motor reverberating pathways. In this case, the pathway in question includes that of the parietal lobe through the frontal lobe to the lenticular nuclei to the thalamus and then to the parietal lobe. Along the way, connections arrive from the red nucleus and from the substantia nigra. This motor reverberating pathway as outlined facilitates graded motor control of the patient's limbs as they move through space. Interruption of that pathway places long motor tracts originating from the midbrain, pons, and medulla to spinal segments in an overactive or hyperactive status.

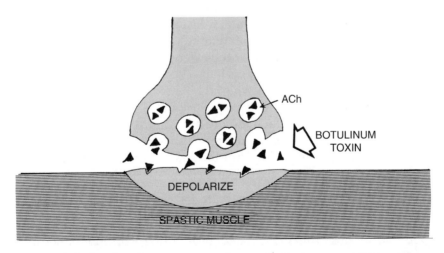

Figure 1.3 Basis of treatment of spasticity by use of botulinum toxin. The normal neuromuscular junction functions by an action potential release of acetylcholine (ACh), which crosses the cleft and attaches to the neural membrane and depolarizes the muscle. In this case, a spastic muscle, is "denervated" by attaching to the presynaptic neuron and blocking the discharge of ACh. (Courtesy of Dr. Rene Cailliet.)

For example, it is difficult to change movement of the limb through space once it has been initiated. The movement will most likely be patterned in synergy.

As a direct consequence of the interruption of this motor pathway and subsequent long-tract overdrive, the ability of the patient to coordinate muscular response is seriously impaired. This patient cannot plan sequential muscular movement through space and also participate in fine motor coordination. Plastic rigidity destroys the patient's capacity for graded motor control.

The limb is only able to be moved in patterns. Major influences generating this central nervous system hyperactive, disordered motor neural control are (1) relative ischemia from small arterioles supplying the nerves, (2) direct irritation from the hemorrhage, and (3) interrupted control of internal body heat and cooling controls. In any case, functional motor dependency will have been produced in transfers, in activities of daily living, and in standing activities and gait.

REFLEXES

Reflexes are not homogenous in their functional effects, though they are relatively easier to monitor. The time they are elicited after the onset of the stroke (ictus) does matter. For example, after ictus, even while deep tendon reflexes cannot be obtained or are equivocal at worst, Hoffmann's reflexes could well be abnormal.[18–22] The Hoffmann's reflex is, moreover, usually present when the bladder is full, and it is usually absent right after the bladder has been emptied. In the early morning when the patient is half asleep, Hoffmann's reflexes are absent, but in mid-afternoon when the patient is at physical therapy, Hoffmann's reflexes are much easier to obtain. Placing the intrinsic muscles of the parietal lobe hand on stretch facilitates it. Hoffmann's and Babinski's reflexes respond in this manner because they are dependent on muscular tone. They can become relatively unremarkable. Even "hard" neurologic signs can become variable under specific circumstances.

Neurologic signs are not absolute but exist only with regard to the full clinical pattern expressed in the environment. It is common for even "hard" signs to appear and disappear during a 24-hour period.[15–18] Hoffmann's and Babinski's reflexes have relatively superficial functional significance. Deep tendon reflexes are expressed using a sensory stimulation (e.g., suddenly stretching a tendon with a hammer) to elicit a muscular control response (e.g., movement of a part of the limb). Hyperreflexic deep tendon reflexes are markers for loss of dynamic sensation of the limb as it moves through space and also for the loss of graded motor control. Therefore, hyperactive deep tendon reflexes in a patient with a hemorrhagic stroke are associated with poor functional use of that limb. These patients will have much more difficulty becoming self-sufficient. They frequently remain functionally dependent.

EFFECT ON REHABILITATION

Even with technologic advances in imaging, monitoring dynamic sensation serially is still an accurate, effective, efficient method of observing how responsive the patient's central nervous system is likely to be to the strain and stress of daily rehabilitation. Studying dynamic sensation initiates a significant chain of phenomena that modifies the patient's rehabilitation potential. For example, observing dynamic sensation frequently through time helps the patient respond to serial, sequential sensations, and then helps the patient to build sequential motor actions. Sequential motor actions at modulated strengths generate functional graded motor control. Dynamic sensation and functional graded motor control will yield progress in fine and gross motor coordination therapy. Fine motor coordination in turn is likely to be associated with advances in cognition, judgment, and discrimination and with significant advances in safe functional outcome.[10,12,20–25] The key evolution is that frequent, organized stimulation of dynamic sensation augments the chances of the patient developing graded motor control. Without dynamic sensation and graded motor control, the parietal lobe hand will not be functional. With it, the patient's grasp and also his or her rehabilitation potential are increased after application to activities of daily living and safe homemaking activities.

REFERENCES

1. Robins M, Baum HM. Incidence. *Stroke* 1981;12(2 Pt 2 Suppl 1)I:45–57.
2. Matsumoto N, *et al*. Natural history of stroke in Minnesota. *Stroke* 1973; 4:20–29.
3. Heyman A, *et al*. Cerebrovascular disease in the bi-racial population of Evans County, Georgia. *Stroke* 1971;2:509–518.
4. Garraway WM, *et al*. The declining incidence of stroke. *N Engl J Med* 1979;300:449–452.
5. Wolf PA, *et al*. Prospective investigations: the Framingham study and the epidemiology of stroke. *Adv Neurol* 1978;19:107–120.
6. Phillips LH II, *et al*. The unchanging pattern of subarachnoid hemorrhage in a community. *Neurology* 1980;30:1034–1040.
7. Kurtzke JF. *Epidemiology of Cerebrovascular Disease*. Berlin: Springer-Verlag, 1969.

8. Hammond PH. The influence of prior instruction to the subject on an apparently involuntary neuromuscular response. *J Physiol (Lond)* 1956;132:17–18P.
9. Hellebrandt FA, *et al*. Tonic neck reflexes in exercises of stress in man. *Am J Phys Med* 1956;35:144.
10. Desmedt JE. *Motor Unit Types, Recruitment and Plasticity in Health and Disease*. Basel, Switzerland: S. Karger, 1981.
11. Dyck PJ. *Peripheral Neuropathy*. Philadelphia: Saunders, 1993.
12. Kaplan CP, Corrigan JD. The relationship between cognition and functional independence in adults with traumatic brain injury. *Arch Phys Med Rehabil* 1994;75:643–647.
13. Kaplan PE. Blink reflex studies and somatosensory cerebral evoked potentials in patients with stroke and aphasia. *EMG Clin Neurophysiol* 1978;18:340–343.
14. Kaplan PE. Blink reflex studies and sensory dysfunction in patients with stroke: the role of dynamic perception. *EMG Clin Neurophysiol* 1979;19:329–334.
15. Kaplan PE, *et al*. The use of the blink reflex in evaluating the patient with stroke and communication disorder. *EMG Clin Neurophysiol* 1977;17:333–338.
16. Kaplan PE, Cerullo L. *Stroke Rehabilitation*. Boston: Butterworths, 1986.
17. Kaplan PE, Materson R. *The Practice of Rehabilitation Medicine*. Springfield, IL: Charles C. Thomas, 1982.
18. Kaplan PE, *et al*. Stroke and brachial plexus injury. *Arch Phys Med Rehabil* 1977;58:415–418.
19. Peachey L. *Handbook of Physiology: Section 10, Skeletal Muscle*. Baltimore: Williams & Wilkins, 1983.
20. Steindler A. *Kinesiology of the Human Body under Normal and Pathological Conditions*. Springfield, IL: Charles C. Thomas, 1955.
21. Sunderland S. *Nerve Injuries and their Repair*. New York: Churchill Livingstone, 1991.
22. Sunderland S. The anatomy and physiology of nerve injury. *Muscle Nerve* 1990;13:771–784.
23. Sunderland S. The anatomic foundation of peripheral nerve repair techniques. *Orthop Clin North Am* 1981;12:245–266.
24. Tyrer JH, Sutherland JM, Eadie MJ. *Exercise in Neurological Diagnosis, third edition*. New York: Churchill Livingstone, 1981.
25. White EL. *Cortical Circuits*. Boston: Birkhauser, 1989.

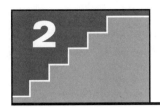

Frontal Lobe Leg

Paul E. Kaplan

In the United States, hemorrhagic strokes represent the single highest contributor to the overall death rate from cerebrovascular disease.[1] Although the contribution of hemorrhagic stroke toward the death rate is not as great as noted in Japan, it is greater than that observed in England and Wales. Hemorrhagic strokes have been studied in smaller, more homogenous groups. Increasing age and hypertension have been identified as major contributing factors to intracerebral hemorrhage.[2] Elevated diastolic blood pressures have been closely associated with transient ischemic attacks and intracerebral hemorrhage.[3] However, most subarachnoid hemorrhages are generated by intracranial aneurysms and arteriovenous malformations.[4–6] Multiple intracranial aneurysms can occur almost 25% of the time.[5,7] Although lifestyle habits (e.g., diet and smoking) do contribute to the overall morbidity and mortality (see Chapter 6), it is clear that genetic factors are also important to the genesis of both hypertension and hemorrhagic stroke. Part of the risk of hemorrhagic stroke is, in effect, built into these patients. Hypertension and diet can be managed and controlled. Smoking can be terminated as a habit. These items represent factors that can be altered or modified. They tend to increase the importance of the primary treating physician's managerial role.

POSTURE OF THE LOWER LIMB

Posture is not only generated by reflexes modifying central nervous system function, but it is also modified by the action of corticospinal tracts.[8,9] Rubrospinal, vestibulospinal, and reticulospinal tracts are organized by spinal segmental level. They could change flexor and extensor muscle tone. Consequently, they alter the ability of the musculoskeletal system to respond to those reflexes that are activated.

Similar to some primitive reflexes, their influences are augmented during periods of extreme stress in normal, intact individuals.

The posture of the lower limb affected by frontal lobe dysfunction (the frontal lobe leg) has also been known for thousands of years. The posture of the frontal lower limb is as follows:

1. The leg is held in extension.
2. The limb is externally rotated.
3. The forefoot is partly plantar flexed.
4. The forefoot is partly supinated.

This posture is essentially based on musculoskeletal hyperactivity of antigravity extensor muscles of the lower limb. Like the parietal lobe hand, the frontal lobe limb is probably caused by necrosis of brain tissue after hemorrhagic strokes, because hemoglobin is cytotoxic. In hemorrhagic strokes, these postures might be evanescent. Neural plasticity is believed to influence the duration of these postures as is the presence of redundant, supernumerary cerebral hemisphere cortical circuits.[10–24] Another factor resides in cells lining the ventricles that can convert to cerebral stem cells, as these cells have the potential to replace lost neural tissue. If either of these factors is functional, neurologic return within the central nervous system would be enhanced. Otherwise, glial scar tissue proliferates and effectively blocks neural regeneration, limiting neurologic return.

Long-tract hyperactivity from the brain stem to lumbosacral spine segments produces hyperactive intrinsic foot muscle contraction. With increased muscular responsiveness of intrinsic foot muscles, a significant external rotation moment is generated throughout the involved lower limb. The plane of action for the knee is changed from the anterior/posterior plane to that of the medial/lateral plane.[10,17–20] Rotation of the plane of action in space obliterates the function of the knee, lengthening that frontal lobe leg.

Extensor hyperactivity, therefore, of the lower limb means that knee flexion, which smooths and buffers gait during stance segments, is not present. As a result, this shift of plane not only lengthens the involved limb, but it also makes it more rigid and less responsive to willed, isolated, volitional motion. Control of that frontal lobe leg is changed from volitional toward patterned movement. The foot is held externally rotated and partially supinated, reducing the medial area of the sole of the foot—surface area that would normally be available for use in weight transfer activities. Consequently, modification of control of motion of the frontal lobe leg makes smooth weight transfer along the sole of that foot difficult.

GAIT ABNORMALITIES

Gait has been described as "controlled falling." To make it even more complex, as we fall, we twist and untwist. Gait is usually rather stable primarily because, as each joint's geometric center moves through space, it contributes to the overall gait stability by moving as little as possible and by keeping the body's center of gravity as low as possible. Consequently, when gait is evaluated, it is examined in stance and swing in six segments: heel strike, midstance, heel off, toe off, midswing, and heel strike. During these six segments, the pelvis femur and tibia shift between medial (inside) and lateral (outside) orientation, as in Figure 2.1.

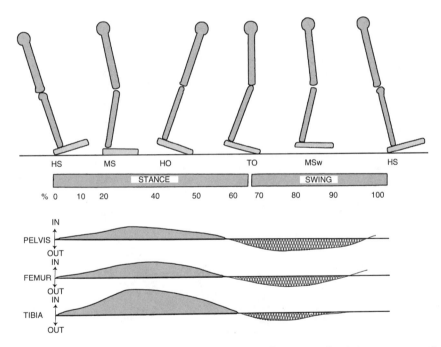

Figure 2.1 Gait cycle. The percentage denotes the increments of a full gait cycle. In this figure, the right leg in one cycle is the heel strike (HS) beginning the stance phase (62%). At HS, the knee is extended (KE). As the body passes over the weight-bearing leg, the knee flexes slightly (KF) to absorb the shock. At midstance (MS, 30%), the knee is fully extended (KE). At heel off (HO, 40%), the knee begins to flex slightly (KF, 50%) and remains flexed through toe off (TO, 62%) when the swing phase begins. The knee remains flexed throughout the swing phase until just before the HS recurs, when the knee re-extends (KE, 100%). (MSw = midswing.) (Reprinted with permission from Cailliet R. *Knee Pain and Disability, second edition*. Philadelphia: F.A. Davis, 1983;154.)

During the stance phase segments, the geometric center of the ankle joint moves through space. The fact that the geometric center is low and moves so conservatively makes the ankles' contribution to gait that much more stable. In that process, the geometric center of the ankle joint delineates arcs as it moves through space (Figure 2.2).

The relative motion of the geometric center of the knee joint through space produces a double pumping or flexion of the knee during stance phase segments. At the same time, the ankle arc patterns are generating ankle plantar flexion (read this motion at least in part as "extension") and ankle dorsiflexion (read this motion at least in part as "flexion"). The coordination of knee flexion/extension and ankle flexion/extension buffers, smooths, and dampens the pathway of the entire body's center of gravity to minimize that body's expenditure of energy during gait (Figure 2.3).

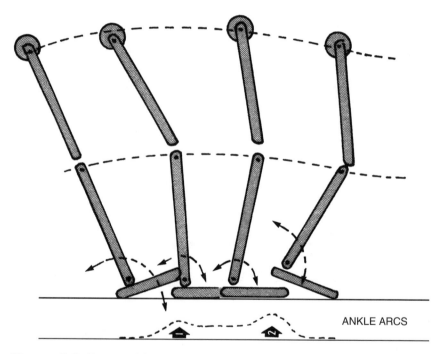

ANKLE ARCS

Figure 2.2 Foot-ankle relationship in gait. Fourth determinant. At heel strike, the ankle is dorsiflexed 90 degrees (and supinated). The level of the ankle rises slightly as the foot goes forward into "flat foot stance." This is followed by the ankle again dorsiflexing as the leg passes over the foot. At push off, the heel rises, giving a second small upward undulation. These small undulations at the ankle are "smoothed out" by simultaneous knee flexion. (Reprinted with permission from Cailliet R. *Foot and Ankle Pain, third edition.* Philadelphia: F.A. Davis, 1997;56.)

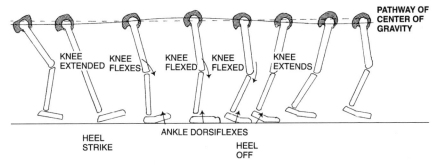

Figure 2.3 Knee flexion during stance phase of gait. Third determinant. The knee is fully extended at heel strike. As the body moves over the center of gravity, the knee flexes slightly to decrease the vertical amplitude of the pathway of the center of gravity. This slight flexion also cushions the impact of the body. The knee re-extends at the end of the stance phase: the heel off. (Reprinted with permission from Cailliet R. *Foot and Ankle Pain, third edition.* Philadelphia: F.A. Davis, 1997;54.)

A direct result of knee-ankle coordination is that during the stance and swing phase segments, the foot/ankle complex dorsiflexes/plantar flexes, supinates/pronates, and internally/externally rotates simultaneously as the lower limbs twist and untwist during gait (Figure 2.4).

Of the six determinants of gait that have been described, three concern the hip, and one each has been designated for the knee and ankle. The sixth gait determinant is precisely the coordination of knee and ankle motion mentioned above. The central feature in a patient with a frontal lobe leg during gait is the absence of smooth twisting and untwisting motion of the lower limb.[17–22] Seamless, buffered winding and unwinding of the lower limb applies the foot to the floor and generates smooth weight transfer along the sole of the foot.

While the lower limb is twisting, internal rotation is driven by large, proximal, pennate hip adductor and flexor musculature, which nearly always are activated together—an activity of type two muscles. During untwisting, however, external rotation is powered by the small, highly leveraged, parallel internal musculature of the foot—an activity initiated by type one muscles but followed by the activation of more proximal and less leveraged type two muscles. To initiate the complex untwisting motion, the body uses a uniquely sophisticated functional musculoskeletal structure located in the sole of the foot. Of the five musculotendinous layers situated on the sole of the foot, each has a variable ratio of fibrous tissue to muscular contractile tissue. Each layer therefore exhibits a special, separate differential contraction velocity.

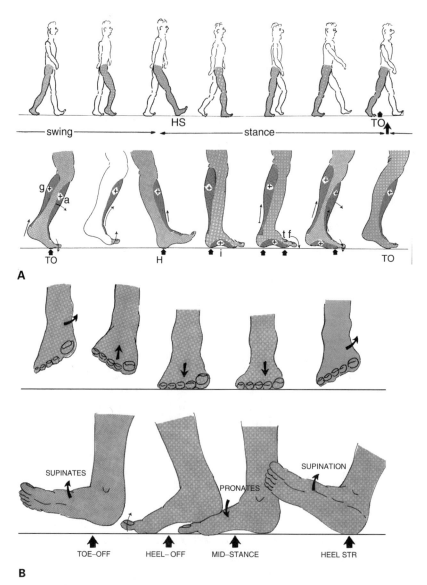

Figure 2.4 A. Coordinated muscular activity during gait to toe off (TO). The gastrocnemius muscle (g) contracts, as does the anterior tibialis (a) to prepare the foot to dorsiflex. At heel strike (HS, H, HEEL STR), only the anterior tibialis contracts, then at midstance, the gastrocnemius contracts to decelerate the forward movement of the body as the plantar muscles contract. At the fifth phase, the gastrocnemius decelerates, and the intrinsic foot muscles (i) and the toe flexors (tf) contract for TO. All this is programmed in the brain for normal, automatic movement. **B**. Role of pronation and supination of the foot during weight transfer from posterior to anterior foot. (Reprinted with permission from Cailliet R. *Foot and Ankle Pain, third edition*. Philadelphia: F.A. Davis, 1997;64.)

These layers are preset at different intrinsic tension states and are therefore made more or less active or controlled by contraction of the extensor digitorum brevis on the dorsum of the foot. These layers are, for example, very active in uphill climb and on uneven surfaces (Figure 2.5).

This detailed, intricate, interactive, and constantly active biofeedback system initiates external rotation, supination, and plantar flexion, effectively lengthening the lower extremity. After a hemorrhagic stroke and subsequent long-tract hyperactivity, this system is usually set at a hyperactive level. The action of these intrinsic muscles is rendered overly responsive to external stimulation. During hyperactivity of the sole of the foot's biofeedback system, winding/unwinding of that foot is interrupted at the height of double stance and at heel-off segments.

The gait type is unique. The knee is vigorously and constantly swung outward in external rotation, supination, and plantar flexion—a circumducted gait. At the two segments mentioned above during the

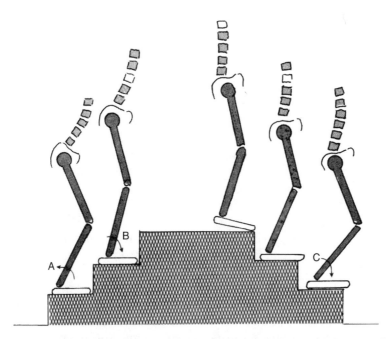

Figure 2.5 Foot-ankle action during stair climbing and descending. As a person climbs stairs, the knee flexes approximately 50%, and the body leans forward. The foot-ankle initially dorsiflexes passively (A) and gradually plantar flexes (B) as the knee extends. In descent, the gastrocnemius soleus decelerates the foot as it dorsiflexes passively (C). (Reprinted with permission from Cailliet R. *Foot and Ankle Pain, third edition.* Philadelphia: F.A. Davis, 1997;65.)

stance phase, this extensor pattern produced by the hyperactive foot actually blocks effective gait. At the height of double stance, the hip and knee extend and the ankle has to flex. At heel off, the hip and knee flex but the normal ankle has to extend. Patients with circumducted gait cannot produce the following gait components:

1. Double knee flexion during the stance phase
2. Coordination of knee and ankle flexion
3. Facilitation of pelvic tilt by functional knee flexion

With three of six gait determinants rendered dysfunctional, the body's center of gravity is displaced by 200% or 300% of normal. The gait activity thus is made less stable, slower, and more expensive in metabolic cost,[10–15,20–22] and the patient will limp. Additionally, the patient's risk of falling is augmented if that patient is in the process of starting, stopping, turning, or being passed by other people. Indeed, during transfer activities using a standing pivot transfer methodology, all of these conditions are met, and the patient will be vulnerable to injury.

SENSATION OF THE LOWER LIMB

Sensory nerves in the foot are far more deeply placed than those of the hand. Consequently, the margin between abnormal and normal two-point discrimination in the foot is so much reduced that two-point discrimination is not nearly as serviceable a determination for dynamic sensation in the foot as it is in the hand.[10,16,19] Stereognosis is still useful, and the procedure can be followed as depicted in Chapter 1. Additionally, the following alternative stereognostic procedure can be followed:

1. Choose objects to be identified. These should include a wooden No. two pencil, a metal key, and a hook cut from soft foam material.
2. Present each object in turn to the patient's normal hand. Have the patient turn it over with his or her fingers while identifying.
3. Have the patient remove shoes, socks, stockings, hose, wrappings, etc. Have the patient place his or her feet on a level surface.
4. Present the objects to the patient's feet, approaching the sole underside of the patient's toes. Have the patient try to turn the objects over with his or her toes, helping to turn them over if needed.

Either stereognostic procedure will establish that patients with a frontal lobe leg have defective dynamic sensation, even if static sensation (e.g., light touch and pin prick) is intact. Right after ictus, dynamic sensation characteristically disappears and usually returns for a brief period (1–2 weeks) only to disappear again. At that point, a patient with a frontal lobe foot will not know where that foot is as he or she moves it through space—in both gait and transfer activities—unless he or she has been trained to monitor that gait visually. In this respect, the frontal lobe foot is exactly comparable to the parietal lobe hand.

Moreover, if the blood supply of both anterior cerebral arteries is impaired, both feet will become frontal lobe feet—a condition termed *cerebral paraplegia*. In this situation, the patient becomes effectively blind to the location of both lower extremities as they move through space. In hemorrhagic stroke syndromes, cerebral paraplegia is still far more common than bilateral middle cerebral artery impairment, even though cerebral paraplegia is often underdiagnosed.[11–16,19,20] When cerebral paraplegia does present, the patient has commonly experienced a fractured hip from a fall, has had total hip arthroplasty, and has not responded to therapeutic gait or transfer activities.

Just as the upper limb can demonstrate a complex regional pain syndrome presentation of hand-shoulder syndrome, the lower limb also has its rotator cuff and can present with a hip-foot syndrome. As with the hand-shoulder syndrome, the hip-foot syndrome usually starts proximally in the shoulder or hip but may be noted distally with dysfunction or pain in the hand or foot. The hip-foot syndrome often presents early after ictus and can quickly acquire a burning pain element and a swollen and discolored foot. With time, the nails become brittle, the hand or foot loses hair, and intrinsic bones of the hand or foot may become osteopenic.

STRENGTH AND TONE OF THE LOWER LIMB

At first flaccid, the tone of the lower limb after ictus usually becomes classically spastic with the characteristic clasp-knife reflex. Spasticity will remain associated with flexion or extension movement patterns until willed, isolated, or volitional activity has been completely restored to the involved joint. Even then, resolution of the spasticity could be incomplete.

One myth is that the spastic limb is therefore strong. It is not strong—control of willed movement has become impaired. Moreover, spasticity also inhibits strength as well as motion. A second myth is that extensor spasticity helps support gait. But at the two strategic points described above, it actually obstructs safe gait and transfer activities. Additionally, during unexpected weight transfers, the clasp-knife characteristic can generate a sudden, reactive flexor reflex—the total collapse of the affected limb. As with the upper limb after ictus, hypertonicity often masks reduced endurance, power, and control or placement capacity. A walk of a longer distance will, in time, often present the patient with the necessity of either an elective rest period or of sudden and rather complete collapse. If the patient has started fatigued, or the conditions were inclement, the time or distance to collapse might not be very long. With higher metabolic costs and blindness of the location of the foot in space, these patients have high insecurity about their mobility capacity—a realistic anxiety.

REFLEXES

Spasticity from stroke syndromes, along with such "hard" neurologic signs as the full Babinski's reflex, are not poured in concrete. When the patient is asleep, his or her bladder is empty, and he or she is relaxed, these signs can become very difficult to elicit.[19–24] When the patient is stressed, his or her bladder or bowel is stretched, and he or she is under the pressure of performance, spasticity, hyperactive deep tendon reflexes, and the Babinski's reflex are floridly present. It is not unusual for two clinicians examining the same patient under different circumstances to elicit vastly differing findings.

Additionally, patients after a hemorrhagic stroke do not necessarily respond well in stressful examination situations. Furthermore, particularly early in patients' acute rehabilitation course after a subarachnoid hemorrhage, hyperactive deep tendon reflexes and abnormal Babinski's reflexes can be present one day and absent the next before they become well established. Many times, Babinski's reflexes are equivocal or partially abnormal. This type of clinical situation often occurs on those days during which the patient is hypertensive, obtunded, and poorly communicative. The combination is part of a clinical pattern of hypertensive encephalopathy. After vigorous treatment with antihypertensive agents, the patient will often respond to the stabilization of his or her blood pressure with regression of abnormal reflexes over the next 7–10 days.

EFFECT ON REHABILITATION

Frontal lobe leg patients are in danger. They experience reduced balance and have little idea where their lower limb is as it moves through space. These patients, therefore, are at a high risk of falling. Usually, these falls follow periods of prolonged inactivity in a semisupine position. During the inactive period, negative calcium and protein metabolic balances have weakened long bones.[17–19] Moreover, after long periods of bed, armchair, or couch rest, as these patients arise, their blood pressures have a tendency to fall, and pulses have a tendency to rise. Blood pressure and pulse regulation is not as effective or efficient. Standing activities lead to light-headedness and vertigo. Walking is no longer a controlled falling process. The patient falls—perhaps multiple times. With those falls come fractures and showers of fat emboli. Complications and sequelae include renal infarcts or failure, cardiac ischemia, thrombotic strokes, or pulmonary emboli. These falls can be lethal.

Even if falls and fractures are prevented by nursing unit safety programs, these patients will probably not do very well in therapy for mobility activities. Absence of dynamic sensation also reduces capacities for sequential motor activities, graded motor contractions, and, ultimately, fine motor coordination and balance. Anxiety generated by the threat of further physical harm can itself become obstructive. Anxiety and anxious depression can control these patients' rate of progress. However, patients with a frontal lobe foot after a hemorrhagic stroke often do respond to patience, to a planned and relaxed approach, and to endless repetition. There is no deadline for these patients if safe progress is desired as the end result. Hope should be cultivated that these patients can become self-sufficient. However, good results take time and much continuous energy and effort.

Outside of a great concentration on physical therapy, amphetamine administration at an early stage after ictus can help reduce the area of cortical necrosis and increase patient concentration. On the other hand, amphetamines can also stress the cardiovascular system and lower the seizure threshold. Delayed heart attacks, coronary artery spasms, seizures, stroke extensions, and new strokes are all unwanted amphetamine sequelae and complications.

REFERENCES

1. Goldberg ID, Kurland LT. Mortality in 33 countries from diseases of the nervous system. *World Neurol* 1962;3:444–462.
2. Furlan AJ, *et al*. The decreasing incidence of primary intracerebral hemorrhage. *Ann Neurol* 1979;5:367–373.
3. Freis ED. Effect of treatment of hypertension on the occurrence of stroke. *Cerebrovasc Dis* 1974;9:133–136.
4. McKissock W, Paine KWE. Subarachnoid hemorrhage. *Brain* 1959;82:356–366.
5. Locksley HB. Report on the Cooperative Study of Intracranial Aneurysms and Subarachnoid Hemorrhage. Section V, Part I. *J Neurosurg* 1966;25:219–239.
6. Pakarinen S. Incidence, aetiology, and prognosis of primary subarachnoid hemorrhage. *Acta Neurol Scand* 1967;29(Suppl 43):1–128.

7. Locksley HB. Report on the Cooperative Study of Intracranial Aneurysms and Subarachnoid Hemorrhage. Section V, Part II. *J Neurosurg* 1966;25:321–368.

8. Snell RS. *Clinical Neuroanatomy for Medical Students.* Boston: Little, Brown, 1987.

9. Kandell ER, Schwartz JH, Jessell TM. *Principles of Neural Science.* Norwalk, CT: Appleton & Lange, 1991.

10. Adams HP Jr. Antithrombolytic therapy for the prevention of recurrent aneurysmal subarachnoid hemorrhage. *Semin Neurol* 1986;5:309–315.

11. Berlowitz DR, *et al.* Inadequate management of blood pressure in a hypertensive population. *New Engl J Med* 1998;339:1957–1963.

12. Del Zoppo GJ. Thrombolytic therapy in cerebrovascular disease. *Stroke* 1988;19:1174–1179.

13. Finn SS, *et al.* Observations on the perioperative management of aneurysmal subarachnoid hemorrhage. *J Neurosurg* 1986;65:48–62.

14. Inman VT, Ralston HJ, Todd F. *Human Walking.* Baltimore: Williams & Wilkins, 1981.

15. Jahss MH. *Disorders of the Foot.* Philadelphia: W.B. Saunders, 1982.

16. Kaplan PE. Blink reflex studies and sensory dysfunction in patients with stroke. *EMG Clin Neurophysiol* 1979;19:329–334.

17. Kaplan PE. The patient with myocardial infarction. *Rehab Med J* 1979;155:213–214.

18. Kaplan PE, *et al.* Calcium balance in paraplegic patients. *Arch Phys Med Rehabil* 1978;59:447–450.

19. Kaplan PE, Kaplan C. Blink reflex. *Arch Phys Med Rehabil* 1980;61:30–33.

20. Murray MP, Drought AB, Kory RC. Walking patterns of normal men. *J Bone Joint Surg* 1964;46A:335–360.

21. Perry J. *Gait Analysis.* Thorofare, NJ: SLACK Inc., 1992.

22. Perry J, *et al.* The determinants of muscle action in the hemiparetic lower extremity. *Clin Orthop* 1978;131:71–89.

23. SHEP Cooperative Research Group. Prevention of stroke by antihypertensive drug treatment in older persons with isolated systolic hypertension: final results of the Systolic Hypertension in the Elderly Program. *JAMA* 1991; 265:3255–3264.

24. Vermeij FH, *et al.* Impact of medical treatment on the outcome of patients after aneurysmal subarachnoid hemorrhage. *Stroke* 1998;29:924–930.

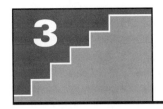

Thalamic Hyperreflexia

Paul E. Kaplan

Although hypertension is the leading cause of hemorrhage into the thalamus, the presence of arteriovenous malformations or aneurysms could also contribute to the overall incidence. As it is, thalamic hemorrhage accounts for 15% of the overall incidence of primary intracerebral hemorrhage.[1] Additionally, thalamogeniculate arteries supplying the thalamus are likely to generate microaneurysms. Although ictus in this area classically brings a distinctive hemisensory deficit pattern associated with a milder hemiparesis, distinctive findings have been identified after hemorrhage into the posterior thalamus.[2] Certainly, ocular findings help with the diagnosis, commonly including convergence-depression syndrome and convergence-retraction nystagmus. In any case, thalamic hemorrhages with thalamic hematomas are often associated with sudden and significant augmentations in intracranial pressure.[3] Increasing intracranial pressure would cause headaches with nausea and vomiting in those affected patients. If the rise of intracranial pressure is large enough, however, it might cause herniation of brain tissue, which would apply compressive pressures directly on the brain stem.[4]

Damage within the thalamus caused by thalamic hemorrhage—especially when lesions have also involved the pyramidal tract—has been associated with absence seizures.[5] These seizures have been typically marked by sudden stops of ongoing actions and lack of responsiveness.[6] In addition, facial clonus and automatic actions have also been observed. Associated with these signs and symptoms have been inhibition associated with gamma-aminobutyric acid activity and then excitation associated with glutamate activity.[5,7] Moreover, the ability of the irritated thalamus to produce hypokinesia and dystonia is illustrated in the application of thalamotomy to treat distal dystonia.[8,9]

The thalamus is strategically positioned within the "interbrain," or diencephalon. It is an older part of the brain than the cerebral hemispheres, which is well-developed in reptiles. The thalami are oval, 4-cm long, and are to be found on either side of the third ventricle.[10–24]

Inferiorly, the thalamus is continuous with the prolongation of the tegmentum and is superior to the hypothalamus. The hypothalamus and thalamus are closely connected, with reverberating neuronal pathway circuits, including the cerebral hemispheres on one hand and the brain stem and spine on the other (Figure 3.1).

Superiorly and medially, the thalamus is separated from the third ventricle by the tela choroidea and the body of the fornix. Moreover, the lateral part of the thalamus forms the floor of the fourth ventricle. The thalamus itself is largely formed by gray matter, but both its lateral and superior surfaces are invested by white matter.[10,21,24] In reptiles, the thalamus became a miniature cerebral hemisphere. In primates, the thalamus became an important relay station between the brain stem/spinal cord and the cerebral hemispheres. Many sensory affective neurons primarily end in the thalamus. One example of strong, selective evolutionary processes is that the thalamus, coordinating sensory data with emotional and motor responses, is central to human fight-or-flight responses (Figure 3.2).

A portion of the basal ganglia layer, thalamus, and midbrain are supplied by a band of small to medium-sized tough arterioles that arise

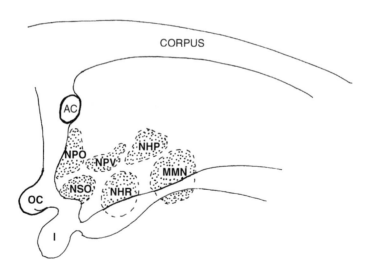

Figure 3.1 Principal nuclei of the hypothalamus. The efferents passing to the thalamus are probably the major routes to the cortex where the sensations are interpreted. (AC = anterior commissure; I = infundibulum; MMN = medial mamillary nucleus; NHP = nucleus preopticus; NHR = nucleus hypothalamus retromedialis; NPO = nucleus preopticus; NPV = nucleus paraventricularis; NSO = nucleus supraopticus; OC = optic chiasma.) (Reprinted with permission from Cailliet R. *Pain: Mechanisms and Management*. Philadelphia: F.A. Davis, 1993;41.)

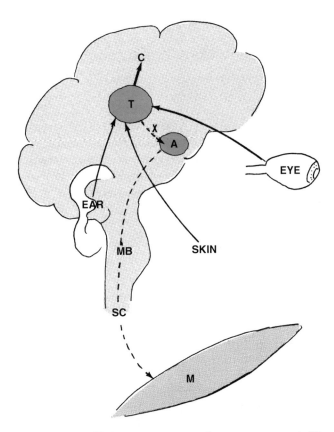

Figure 3.2 Fight-or-flight response to fear: a concept. The current pathway of visual (from eye), auditory (from ear), and tactile (from skin) impulses to the thalamus then the cortex (C), where memory invokes a neuromuscular response (*dark arrows*). In a newer concept (see text), the impulses go from the thalamus (T) to the amygdala (A) then directly (path X) to the midbrain (MB), where neuromuscular patterns proceed via the spinal cord (SC) to the effector muscles (M). (Courtesy of Dr. Rene Cailliet.)

proximally from the posterior cerebral arteries near its origin at the circle of Willis. These smaller arteries, therefore, receive the jet stream–directed arterial blood flow from the posterior circulation of the central nervous system (CNS) at an overlap area with the anterior circulation. In sum, the thalamus can receive connections from any part of the CNS and receives preferential blood supply so that it can, even under unfavorable circumstances, receive sensory data and coordinate emotional and motor responses.

Structurally, the thalamus has become adapted to its special functions. Internally, the thalamus is divided by a vertical lamina of white matter in a Y shape. The anterior and medial nuclei groups are the older part of the organ. The anterior thalamus has close connections with the limbic lobe system and especially with the hippocampus. The thalamus is a vital part of the limbic reverberatory circuit for emotional response. The medial group has close connections with the corpus striatum. The thalamus is thus also a vital part of coordinating sequential motor response. The ventral nuclear group is a vital and strategic relay system for the sensory somatic system, whereas the lateral group is in the same strategic position with regard to the motor, or muscular, system. Sensory data are gathered, and motor response is organized.

The lateral and ventral groups are laminated functionally by spinal neural segments, and both are well connected to long tracts from the basal ganglia and midbrain to the pons, medulla, and spinal cord segments.[10,21,24] Through its extensive midbrain connections, the thalamus has reciprocal connections with the cerebellum. Therefore, any neural impulse traveling through the brain stem caudally or cranially would also be modified and characterized through its impact with the thalamus. This relay station cannot be bypassed.

SENSATION

The midbrain portion of the brain stem receives sensory impulses from the peripheral nervous system and from other special sensory and biofeedback stations, and transmits those impulses to the thalamus and cerebellum, providing afferent input for coordination mentioned above (Figure 3.3).

In particular, the midbrain sends primary and connective-secondary, facilitative, and inhibitive neuronal tracts to and from thalamic nuclei. These nuclei in turn send new neuronal connections to and from the cerebral hemispheres. From the midbrain to the thalamus to the cerebral hemispheres, the connections are dense, varied, and reciprocal (Figure 3.4).

When the CNS is stressed by hypertension, the lenticulostriate arterial system supplying the basal ganglionic area is so placed that it is subjected to the full force of the blood pressure without alleviation. Additionally, that blood pressure is itself controlled by the sympathetic nervous system (Figure 3.5).

It is not surprising that the sympathetic nervous system is frequently involved in hemorrhagic stroke syndromes either alone or, more frequently, as part of a complex clinical syndrome. After a thalamic hemorrhage, the patient will have a deep, visceral, aching emotional feeling associated with intensely and explosively burning pain in the contralateral half of the body. This special emotional feeling is due to the

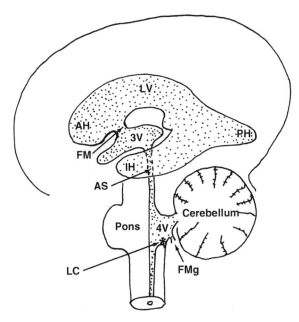

Figure 3.3 Ventricular system of the brain. A schematic illustration of the ventricular system of the brain containing the spinal fluid. (AH = anterior horn; AS = aqueduct of Sylvius; FM = foramen of Monro; FMg = foramen of Magendie; IH = inferior horn; LC = site of locus ceruleus neurons; LV = lateral ventricles; PH = posterior horn; 3V = third ventricle; 4V = fourth ventricle.) (Reprinted with permission from Cailliet R. *Pain: Mechanisms and Management.* Philadelphia: F.A. Davis, 1993;35.)

many direct and indirect connections between the thalamus as the sensory receptor and its position as part of the limbic system (Figure 3.6).

Accompanying the particularly distressing feeling described previously and its associated burning pain is also a mild sensory loss over that same side, but the sensory loss is mild enough in relation to the strong pain and disturbing feeling that it might be ignored. The full medical syndrome is termed *Dejerine-Roussy syndrome*.[10,13,19] The pain and discomfort are made worse by any number of adverse experiences (e.g., negative emotional feelings, hostile environments [art, music, or furnishings], and innocuous but unwelcome types of unexpected tactile stimulations). It has long been noted that position sensation was lost early in the syndrome and also relatively completely. In fact, dynamic sensation is also lost early after ictus and is profound, even when static sensation is only partially abnormal. Even when static sensation returns, dynamic sensation usually does not.

The differential diagnosis is important, and it includes complex regional pain syndromes and reflex sympathetic dystrophy syndromes

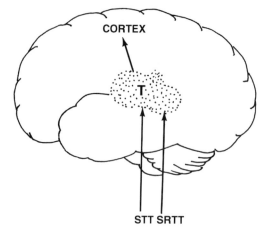

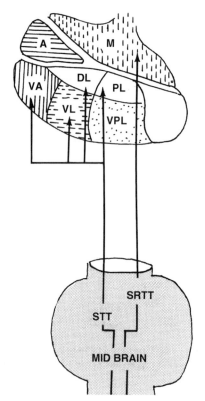

Figure 3.4 Thalamic pathways. The thalamus (T) is a large ovoid gray mass located on either side of the third ventricle. The anterior tubercle (A) is thin and lies close to the midline (M). The posterior portion is known as the *pulvinar*. From the cord, the ascending pathways that connect to the thalamus divide within the midbrain. They include the spinoreticulothalamic tract (SRTT) to the medial aspect of the thalamus and the spinothalamic tracts (STTs). They go directly to the lateral, ventral, and caudal regions. From the thalamus, the pathways ascend to the cortex to as-yet-unknown areas of "representation." (DL = dorsolateral; PL = posterolateral; VA = ventro anterior; VL = ventro lateral; VPL = ventroposterolateral.) (Reprinted with permission from Cailliet R. *Pain: Mechanisms and Management.* Philadelphia: F.A. Davis, 1993;9.)

such as hand-shoulder syndrome or hip-foot syndrome. With thalamic pain, elbow and knee sensation is abnormal. With reflex sympathetic dystrophy, the elbow and knee are spared. The distribution of thalamic pain is also similar to that often noted in a thrombotic stroke

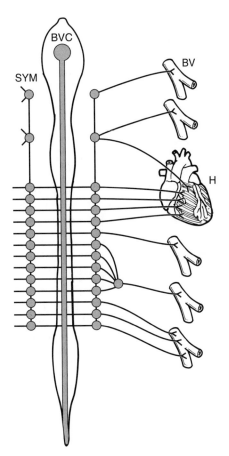

Figure 3.5 Sympathetic nervous system control of the circulation. The autonomic nervous system (SYM) controls the vasomotor system: the blood vessels (BVs) and the heart (H). At the upper aspect of the autonomic nervous system, the vasomotor center (BVC) is located. (Courtesy of Dr. Rene Cailliet.)

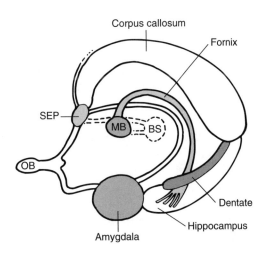

Figure 3.6 Principal connections of the limbic system. Numerous other structures are not shown. (BS = brain stem; MB = mamillary body; OB = olfactory bulb; SEP = septum anterior thalamus.) (Modified from MacLean PD. Psychosomatic disease and the visceral brain. *Psychosom Med* 1949;11:338, as shown in: Chusid JG [ed], *Correlative Neuroanatomy and Functional Neurology.* Los Altos, CA: Lang, 1970;13.)

involving the cerebral hemispheres, but the presence of the intense and troubling pain-feeling combination should indicate that thalamic pain is present.[10-14]

The differential diagnosis, however, of these three pain syndromes could be difficult, as the full syndromes are only partially expressed or may seem mixed. In addition, a hemorrhagic stroke could affect two or more areas of the CNS at the same time.[10-13,19,24] With the advent of scanning technology, it is evident that often both cerebral and thalamic areas of hemorrhagic stroke are present in patients with multiple strokes. The clinical evolution of the syndrome is not so much from cerebral stroke to a hand-shoulder syndrome complication but from combined, complex stroke syndromes to a thalamic pain residual. The full evolution of the pain syndrome should be observed in these patients over time. This clinical situation is especially evident in patients with malignant hypertension. Patients with hemorrhagic strokes used to die from complications of their relentless hypertensive disease. Now, when patients with aggressive hypertensive cardiovascular complications have been successfully medically managed with antihypertensive medication, they experience morbidity from more than one stroke.

Scanning technology has allowed the association to be made between thalamic lesions and a wide variety of mild to moderate cognitive deficits. Frequently, related deficits include aphasia, memory loss, dementia, and other specific cognitive deficits associated with strategically placed thalamic lesions.[12-19] In any one patient, judgmental and discriminative cognitive dysfunction could be generated by thalamic lesions. More correlative anatomic and metabolic studies are currently in progress.

Dominant thalamic lesions have been associated with deficits in spoken language. Reports of deficits in written language have generally also observed thalamic along with other basal ganglia lesions. Aphasia can be observed after hemorrhage into the dominant thalamus that is not limited to paraphasia, reduced verbal output, minimally reduced repetition, and impaired comprehension. Behavioral dysfunction also associated with thalamic lesions includes reduced ambition, inhibition, judgment, motivation, and increased apathy—the typical "frontal lobe syndrome."[21-23] This clinical syndrome has also been observed in brain tumors, severe traumatic brain injuries, and in CNS vasculitis or infections. It can be caused by bilateral thalamic pathology as well as by bilateral frontal lobe lesions.

Behavioral deficits in these patients, however, are also associated with cognitive deficits (e.g., reduced attention span, reduced long-term memory storage, and reduced long-term memory retrieval). These deficits can be exacerbated by depressive and anxiety responses. Consequently, patients with thalamic lesions may be less able to follow complex directions under stress. Therapy for these patients in a gymnasium setting is often difficult because of the distracting, noisy conditions. In most clinical settings, however, behavioral deficits are present in elderly, hypertensive patients with more than one stroke syndrome and broad, widespread memory impairments.

WAVES OF INVOLVEMENT

The evolution of a hemorrhagic thalamic stroke through time is also a large part of the overall deficit. It is not unusual for these patients to be neurologically unstable, mute, or delirious at an early stage after ictus. Many of these seemingly dense deficits do resolve but not necessarily at an even rate. Instead, some movement toward recovery is often arrested or even followed by some regression.[10–16] During the regressive periods, sensation deficits and pain can become more prominent than during periods of initial recovery. Although the overall progress over time is frequently positive, at any one moment in time the patient could present with a relatively progressive cognitive deficit. But the overall shape of recovery is often like an inimitable series of gradually improving short/long sinusoidal waves—individual and unique. It is therefore important for the clinician to become familiar with each patient's pattern.

LACUNA ASSOCIATIONS

The same hypertensive hemorrhage that generates thalamic syndrome can also produce lacuna strokes. Pure motor or sensory deficits are noted, with involvement of the contralateral internal capsule. With time, these occasionally severe deficits often resolve.[20] Early, however, in the patient's course after ictus, these deficits might also leave the patient less neurologically stable, more functionally dependent, and physically deconditioned. Although the overall prognosis for functional recovery is excellent, early metabolic demands associated with mobilization can fall on a CNS still recovering from a hemorrhagic stroke. Therefore, the course of rehabilitation right after ictus in these patients is commonly rocky. These patients require time to heal. If these patients are not allowed to fully and completely stabilize their neurologic presentations as inpatients, many will be given undeservedly poor rehabilitation capacity evaluations. Time is an ally. If these patients are allowed to fully neurologically stabilize, they will become stronger and their neurologic deficits will spontaneously resolve. Consequently, time spent on care and observation of these patients under quiet, supportive, and friendly inpatient conditions is usually well repaid by spectacular clinical functional recoveries during outpatient therapy after discharge.

EFFECT ON REHABILITATION

Rehabilitation potential in thalamic hemorrhage patients is best determined early in the rehabilitative program. To construct an accurate rehabilitation outlook, the physician should be sensitive to these patients' resources, strengths, and weaknesses. Additionally, restoration of function is also one of the consistently useful methods of treating thalamic pain. However, these patients do not necessarily easily accept—much less welcome—therapy, as they fear that any disturbance will increase their pain. Moreover, modalities, acupuncture, transcutaneous nerve stimulation, functional electric stimulation, and neuromuscular re-education have all been used to restore clinical function and reduce pain. There is no one therapeutic "magic bullet" that cures thalamic hemorrhage. Instead, effective, efficient patient management is required. Patients require responsive, calm, supportive, yet accurate observation and intervention.

Treatments should be customized to each patient's rehabilitation potential and periodically reviewed to be effective. Therapy is not necessarily popular. Elderly patients will be hard pressed to maintain positive attitudes during physical and occupational therapy with the stress of pain, weakness, nausea, and embarrassment. The fact that most therapists are younger than these patients does not help. Younger patients are not necessarily easier to treat and often demand the reassurance of a direct, rapid regimen that is guaranteed to produce self-sufficiency fast. In each case, the team should discuss these strains in a beneficial, confidential milieu with enough time appropriated so that each stress is identified and understood. It should be stated that much, including rating functional gains, needs to be done, but if these stresses are not confronted, they will grow and obstruct rehabilitation.

On one hand, these patients at times require intensive inpatient therapy over longer time periods for the clinician/patient team to generate significant functional improvement. On the other hand, rapid improvements, including great advances in safe self-care and mobility, can be realistic for any patient. One key to team success is perpetual and customized team building. The team should place its energy, spirit, and enthusiasm into identifying, discussing, and resolving the stresses and strains of the rehabilitation of thalamic hemorrhage patients. With harmony, agreement, and purpose, no matter how difficult the patient or the problems, the rehabilitation will make significant progress toward its functional goals.

REFERENCES

1. Jones EF, *et al*. Proximal aortic atheroma. *Stroke* 1995;26:218–224.
2. Hirose G, *et al*. The syndrome of posterior thalamic hemorrhage. *Neurology* 1985;35:998–1002.
3. Kase CS, Caplan LR. *Intracerebral Hemorrhage*. Boston: Butterworths, 1994.
4. Barnett HJ, *et al*. *Stroke*. New York: Churchill-Livingstone, 1992.
5. Snead OC. Basic mechanisms of generalized absence seizures. *Ann Neurol* 1995;35:146–157.
6. Gastaut H, Broughton R. *Epileptic Seizures*. Springfield, IL: Charles C. Thomas, 1972.
7. Wyllie E. *The Treatment of Epilepsy*. Baltimore: Williams & Wilkins, 1997.
8. Cardoso F, *et al*. Outcome after stereotactic thalamotomy for dystonia and hemiballismus. *Neurosurgery* 1995;36:501–508.
9. Jancovic J, Tolosa E. *Parkinson's Disease and Movement Disorders*. Baltimore: Williams & Wilkins, 1998.
10. Aminoff MJ, Greenberg DA, Simon RP. *Clinical Neurology*. Stamford, CT: Appleton & Lange, 1996.
11. Besson JM, Guilbaud G, Peschanski M. *Thalamus and Pain*. New York: Elsevier Science, 1987.
12. Brown GG, Kieran S, Patel S. Memory functioning following a left medial thalamic hematoma. *J Clin Exp Neuropsychol* 1989;11:206–218.
13. Caplan LF, *et al*. Lateral thalamic infarcts. *Arch Neurol* 1988:45:959–965.
14. Castaigne P, *et al*. Paramedian thalamic and midbrain infarcts. *Ann Neurol* 1981;10:127–148.
15. Crosson B. *Subcortical Functions in Language and Memory*. New York: The Guilford Press, 1992.
16. Dusoir H, *et al*. The role of diencephalic pathology in human memory disorder. *Brain* 1990;113:1695–1706.
17. Graff-Radford NR, *et al*. Diencephalic amnesia. *Brain* 1990;113:125.
18. Malamut BL, *et al*. Memory in a case of bilateral thalamic infarction. *Neurology* 1992;42:163–169.
19. Purpura DP, Yahr MD. *The Thalamus*. New York: Columbia University Press, 1966.
20. Sacco RL, *et al*. Selective proprioceptive loss from a thalamic, lacuna stroke. *Stroke* 1987;18:1160–1163.
21. Schmitt FO, *et al*. *The Neurosciences*. New York: Rockefeller University Press, 1970.
22. Speedie LJ, Heilman KM. Amnestic disturbance following infarctions of the left dorsomedial nucleus of the thalamus. *Neuropsychology* 1982;20:597–604.
23. Von Cramon DY, Hebel N, Schuri U. A contribution to the anatomical basis of thalamic amnesia. *Brain* 1985;108:993–1008.
24. Warwick R, Williams PL. *Gray's Anatomy*. Philadelphia: W.B. Saunders, 1973.

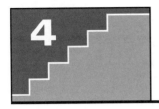

Decorticate Presentation

Paul E. Kaplan

The truly basic or "primitive" postural reflexes cannot usually be studied in intact, functioning, normal adults or animals except under conditions of extreme stress or catastrophic disease, or after the application of special scientific techniques.[1] In animals, that condition is usually met after delivering large brain stem lesions.[2] Sherrington produced decerebrate rigidity in cats after completely transecting the brain stem caudal to the red nucleus.[3] Another method is to study normal pediatric human development, human development in normal children, and development in patients with such disorders as the different types of cerebral palsy.[4] For example, during the development of normal infants, flexor tone of the infant's arms and legs is noted at birth and is masked at 4 and 5 months, respectively.[5] This flexor posture for all four limbs does coincide with the most minimal contribution from the cortex of the infant's cerebral hemispheres.[6,7] The next logical step would be to associate decorticate status with a completely flexor posture. These findings have had significant therapeutic implications, as many of the neuromuscular therapeutic exercise programs applied to both children with cerebral palsy and also to adults after the onset of stroke disorders depend on the facilitation or inhibition of these primary postural presentations, which themselves are the result of spinal, brain stem, and basal ganglion level reflexes.[8–10]

POSTURE

This chapter might just as well be called "the totally reflexive patient." It presents the effects of a hemorrhagic stroke that has affected both cerebral hemispheres.[11–25] As part of the full syndrome, higher cognitive functions are not demonstrated. These patients initially survive by instinct. Later, as a response to intense classical conditioning, some basic procedures seem to be repeated or "learned." This clinical condition is much more frequent than supposed. It can be generated by at least three mechanisms. The first is by direct extension of the hemorrhage. Another is at the period of cerebral hemisphere hypotension and shock that commonly follows ictus. The third is due to the space-consuming nature of the original hemorrhage within the confined space of the skull. Central nervous system hemorrhage presents much as a brain tumor does.

After ictus, for a variable period, the cerebral cortex of both hemispheres often goes into shock and ceases to function.[14-16] During this period, one of two postures is noted. Decerebrate posture is well known. During decerebrate posture, the limbs of the body present in total extension. Decorticate posture is much less well known. During decorticate posture, the limbs of the body present in total flexion—the fetal position (Figure 4.1).

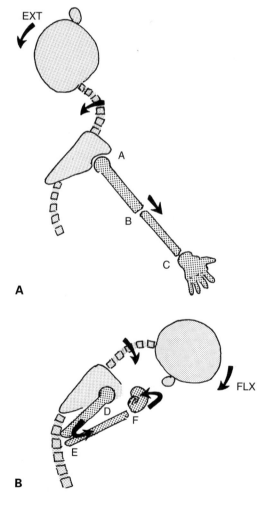

Figure 4.1 A. The extensor (EXT) pattern of the upper extremity in neck extension. **B.** Flexion (FLX) of the upper extremity on neck flexion. (A = shoulder; B = elbow; C = wrist; D = shoulder flexed; E = elbow flexed; F = wrist and fingers flexed.) (Reprinted with permission from Cailliet R. *The Shoulder in Hemiplegia.* Philadelphia: F.A. Davis, 1980;57.)

The clinical presentation of these patients can become complex. With shock of the cerebral cortex, other brain stem reflexes and those involving the basal ganglion level become clinically hyperreflexic. Many times, these patients present in symmetric tonic neck reflex posture. When this postural reflex occurs, the neck is flexed forward, the arms flexed, and the legs extended. One complication of the symmetric tonic neck reflex posture is that the patient has severe difficulty maintaining seating in a wheelchair. Symmetric tonic neck reflex posture has been confused with decorticate posture. Another posture often noted is the asymmetric tonic neck reflex, in which the head is turned toward one side. If toward the left, the patient's left extremities are extended, and the right extremities are flexed.

Both the symmetric and asymmetric tonic neck reflexes are brain stem–releasing postural reflexes. They have direct and indirect functional consequences, as they both complicate bed mobility of the patient. All of these postural reflexes were originally described in patients with deep closed-eye coma, as they have made care of the patient with closed-eye coma more demanding. They are also present, however, in patients with open-eye coma, post-traumatic amnesia, or post-ictal amnesia.

STRENGTH AND TONE

Muscular tone is enhanced at an early stage in decorticate presentation and has a plastic character, as resistance to movement is continuous and smooth with range of motion. When a limb is moved through space, it is moved in flexor or extensor patterns after stimulation as part of a spinal segmental reflex. Although precise, volitional limb placement is not observed, these patterns can be used to train the patient to perform such functional activities as feeding, but millions of repetitions are required to generate the new brain stem reflex neural loops. When the spinal cord remains intact, however, the patient's muscle tone augmentation can be intense, and this densely elevated muscular tone could block functional progress.

As patient response to even one-step direction is not consistent, strength determination is variable but usually seems reduced in all limbs. Movements are, however, often delayed and slow.[11,17–19] On one hand, application of medications usually used to treat Parkinson's disease speeds up these movements somewhat. On the other hand, difficult-to-treat athetoid movements have also been observed in these patients. Generally, what strength remains cannot easily be modified, and fine motor coordination is usually deficient. The combination of muscular rigidity and slowness of response makes daily care activities and bed mobility activities much more difficult. If a given motor activity was one avoided by the patient before stroke, resistance is that much greater, and fine and gross motor coordination harder to treat.

FRONTAL RELEASE SIGNS

When both frontal lobes of the cerebral hemispheres fail to function, a number of reflexes become clinically hyperreflexic. These include the snout, jaw, and palmomental reflexes. They are also clinically prominent. Nonetheless, there is only a relatively small amount of research literature regarding the prognostic value of these release signs. Generally, they have been described in clinical situations in which both cerebral hemispheres have been subjected to a significant insult.[17-20] However, release signs are frequently apparent in the decorticate patient even after the patient's eyes are open and he or she has become responsive. When release signs are present, the patient, with eyes open, still cannot appropriately smile or socialize. Release signs are not usually present if one of the frontal lobes is functional, as with other truly unilateral cerebral lesions. Release signs include

1. The plantar grasp reflex: Presents with toe flexion/adduction after sole stimulation.
2. The palmar grasp reflex: Presents with finger flexion after palmar stimulation.
3. The palmomental reflex: Presents with chin muscle contraction after palmar stimulation.
4. The glabellar reflex: Presents with persistent blinking after repeated glabellar tapping.
5. Suck and snout reflexes: Exhibited after lip stimulation, and the patient might also root toward the direction of the stimulation.

As with most neurologic signs, these reflexes are not equally evident at all points of the day. They are usually easier to elicit early in the morning when the patient is only half awake and relaxed. They become more difficult to elicit with the patient fully awake, tense, and under stress. These signs, in fact, constitute an informal positron emission tomography scan, as their presence is consistent with bilateral, widespread cortical lesions and with a decorticate presentation.

PSEUDOBULBAR SIGNS AND SYMPTOMS

In the presence of bilateral cortical lesions, the basal ganglionic areas of the brain are also released, as noted above. The result is termed *pseudobulbar palsy syndrome.* It is frequently present in a reflexive patient, but this syndrome is usually not obvious until the patient is subject to great stress, anxiety, or panic.[11-13,21-25] Pseudobulbar palsy syndrome includes

1. Dysarthria
2. Dysphagia
3. Emotional lability

The crying frequently exhibited with this syndrome does not have a sad emotion behind it, but is an expression of the stressful situation the patient is experiencing. Laughing is noted less commonly and is also generated by stress or anxiety—not by joy. Indeed, communication is not consistent or appropriate with many of these patients. They become frustrated and angry. Both communication and swallow deficits make feeding activities difficult and unsafe.

EFFECT ON REHABILITATION

The diagnosis of a reflexive patient can be made when the physician enters the room. The patient will posture, be emotionally labile, and present release-type reflexes. More to the point, these patients do not have insight, higher judgmental or cognitive functions, or appropriate socialization capacities. These patients are not able to smile and appropriately contribute socially. In addition, they present with difficulties concerning safe bed mobility, transfer, and feeding activities. They, therefore, represent considerable burdens to adequate nursing care and have increased chances of hurting the staff, other patients, or themselves. As their insight is so baseline, they would not probably be able to fully appreciate how well they have been helped. These are also the most defenseless patients—at risk for complications or sequelae as a result of unsatisfactory care. With intensive rehabilitative nursing care and therapy, these patients can make significant gains in feeding, transfers, and bed mobility. However, the amount of functional rated return measured by the team will probably be relatively small when compared to the cost. Without that intensive rehabilitative care, however, morbidity and mortality of this group of patients are accelerated.

What is the general nature of that intensive rehabilitation program? The details of the therapeutic prescription vary from region to region in the United States. An intensive inpatient rehabilitation program usually includes

1. Repetition: Millions of times for even a simple movement.
2. Calm, controlled, individual therapy in a relaxed, warm, steady, and supportive environment.
3. Much time and patience are required by the rehabilitation team, the patient, and friends and family.
4. Objectives should be kept modest and realistic at all times. A record of success is a valuable portion of the rehabilitative program.

REFERENCES

1. Nashner LM. Adaptation of human movement to altered environments. *Trends Neurosci* 1982;5:358–361.
2. Brodal P. *Motor Systems.* New York: Oxford, 1992.
3. Sherrington C. *The Integrative Action of the Nervous System.* New Haven, CT: Yale University Press, 1947.
4. McGraw MB. *Neuromuscular Maturation of the Human Infant.* New York: Hafner, 1963.
5. Paine RS, *et al.* Evolution of postural reflexes in normal infants and in the presence of chronic brain syndromes. *Neurology* 1964;1036–1041.
6. Prechtl HFR. *Child Neurology and Cerebral Palsy. Clinics Dev Med No 2.* London: Spastics Society, 1960.
7. Connolly K. *Mechanisms of Motor Skill Development.* New York: Academic Press, 1970.
8. Fay T. Basic considerations regarding neuromuscular and reflex therapy. *Spas Q* 1954;29:327–336.
9. Held R, Hein A. Movement produced stimulation in the development of usually guided behavior. *J Comp Physiol Psychol* 1963;56:872–876.
10. Kottke FJ. *Neurophysiologic Therapy for Stroke.* New Haven: E. Licht, 1975.
11. Andrews BT, *et al.* The effects of intracerebral hematoma location on the risk of brainstem compression and outcome. *J Neurosurg* 1988;69:518–522.
12. Benson DF. *Aphasia, Alexia, Agraphia.* New York: Churchill Livingstone, 1979.
13. Brust JCM. Vascular dementia is underdiagnosed. *Arch Neurol* 1988; 45: 799–801.
14. Caronna JJ, Simon RP. The comatose patient. *Int Anesthesiol Clin* 1979;17:3–18.
15. Feldman ME, Sahrmann S. The decerebrate state in the primate. *Arch Neurol* 1971;25:517–525.
16. Fisher CM. The neurological examination of the comatose patient. *Acta Neurol Scand* 1969;Suppl 36:4–56.
17. Grindal AB, Suter C, Martinez AJ. Alpha pattern coma. *Ann Neurol* 1977; 1:371–377.
18. Iragui VJ, McCutchen CB. Physiologic and prognostic significance of "alpha coma." *J Neurol Neurosurg Psychiatry* 1983;46:632–638.
19. Kennard C, Illingworth R. Persistent vegetative state. *J Neurol Neurosurg Psychiatry* 1995;59:347–348.

20. McNealy DE, Plum FP. Brainstem dysfunction with supratentorial mass lesions. *Arch Neurol* 1962;7:10–32.
21. Multi-Society Task Force on PVS. Medical aspects of the persistent vegetative state. *New Engl J Med* 1994;330:1499–1508,1572–1579.
22. Nielsen JM. *Agnosia, Apraxia, Aphasia: Their Value in Cerebral Localization*. New York: Hafner, 1962.
23. Plum FP, Posner JB. *Diagnosis of Stupor and Coma*. Philadelphia: F.A. Davis, 1980.
24. Posner JB. The comatose patient. *JAMA* 1975;232:1313–1314.
25. Tatemichi TK. How acute brain failure becomes chronic. *Neurology* 1990; 40:1652–1659.

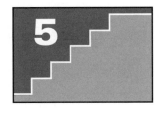

Deficits of the Posterior Circulation of the Central Nervous System

Paul E. Kaplan

When patients were studied who had acquired traumatic brain injuries and had died in automobile accidents, diffuse axonal degeneration was observed.[1] Diffuse axonal degeneration can also be noted in other central nervous system (CNS) injuries. For example, this same phenomenon has been studied in patients with acquired cervical spinal cord injuries.[2,3] Although this condition has been noted in traumatic brain injuries acquired in high-speed motor vehicle accidents when the patients have lost consciousness,[4,5] in those patients with spinal cord injuries, no cervical displacement has been demonstrated. Anatomically, long tracts within the CNS appear to be susceptible, and, microscopically, other features are similar to wallerian-type degeneration.[6] Wallerian degeneration can be found after physical interruptions (e.g., axonotmesis). It also often can be found after disruption of vascular supply.[6–8] Long-tract involvement is also common after vascular disruption.[7–9] It is not surprising that a frequent site of diffuse axonal degeneration is the mesencephalic-pontine junction in proximity to the superior cerebellar peduncles.[10] This finding provides witness to the CNS devastation observed after the vascular disruption of hemorrhagic stroke.

CHARACTERIZATION OF DEFICITS OF POSTERIOR CIRCULATION

The "anterior" circulation to the CNS includes the blood supply from the carotid arteries through the circle of Willis to the cerebral hemispheres.[11–27] The "posterior" circulation, therefore, includes the blood supply from the vertebral and basilar arteries to the brain stem, midbrain, cerebellum, and basal ganglion areas of the CNS. There is an overlap area where the posterior circulation supplies posterior aspects of the circle of Willis.[19,25] In either case, blood flow is thus forcefully directed. Although the capacity exists for these two circulations to mix within the circle of Willis, these two circulations are jet directed toward different locations and commonly do not mix.

This laminar flow does differentiate the two systems. The dynamic structure of the two systems is different. The anterior system facilitates blood volume, and the posterior facilitates pressure. Consequently, it is the posterior circulation that is more vulnerable to hypertensive stress. The posterior system is more thoroughly damaged by hemorrhagic strokes. The characteristic hallmarks of deficits of posterior circulation are crossed sensory and motor abnormalities. As a result, after hemorrhage within the areas supplied by the posterior circulation, motor weakness or ataxia is often ipsilateral, and sensation deficits are contralateral. Of all of the arteries of the posterior circulation, the arteries most commonly affected—and by a 4 to 1 ratio compared to all others combined—are the posterior inferior cerebellar arteries. Hemorrhage of these arteries into the medulla generates Wallenberg's syndrome as outlined below.

1. In Wallenberg's syndrome, ipsilateral facial palsy is combined with contralateral sensation deficits.
2. If the medial branch of the artery is involved, nystagmus is prominent.
3. If the lateral branch is involved (the classic Wallenberg's syndrome), gait ataxia (with special involvement of the ipsilateral limb), meiosis, dysconjugate gaze palsy, and dysarthria may be observed.[19,20,25]
4. Vertigo and ataxia are present in any case.

Frequently, the full syndrome is not expressed. Recent advances in magnetic resonance imaging technology have aided in the differential diagnosis of Wallenberg's syndrome. It is easier to detect the lesions that generate much of this clinical presentation (i.e., intraparenchymal hemorrhage, intracranial aneurysms, and arteriovenous malformations).

SENSATION

Pin prick, temperature, and dynamic sensation deficits of the contralateral half of the body are most often observed in deficits of the posterior circulation. The sensory loss is usually partial, not very dense, and might incompletely recover with time. Although inconvenient, the loss is not similar to that noted in Chapters 1 and 2 for the parietal lobe hand and the frontal lobe foot or as intensive.

Depending on the involved artery and also on the area of the brain stem supplied, these sensory losses will be accompanied by ipsilateral cranial nerve deficits. Cranial nerve deficits usually provide the clearest indications of the true location of the hemorrhagic stroke. Indeed, cranial nerve deficits can be so remarkable that the relatively modest crossed sensory loss is overlooked.[12,14,20,25,26] This dichotomy generates a situation in which these types of strokes can be underdiagnosed, particularly if they are mixed with strokes involving the cerebral hemispheres. The reality is that a high index of suspicion is helpful.

Until recently, brain scan technology was much less effective in evaluating areas supplied by the posterior circulation than it was in evaluating areas supplied by the anterior circulation.[16,22–27] The application of evoked potential electrodiagnosis (i.e., auditory-evoked potentials, visual-evoked potentials, and somatosensory-evoked potentials) helped those clinicians who were already aware of the differential diagnosis.[24] Careful and consistent serial neurologic evaluation is still the necessary foundation for subsequent patient care. Because the limb itself is not completely blind as it moves through space, sensory re-education techniques have been effective with these patients.

CRANIAL NERVE DEFICITS

The following cranial nerve deficits indicate the level of the brain stem affected by the hemorrhagic stroke[11–15]:

1. Lesions of the medulla usually involve cranial nerves IX through XII, leading to the observed dysphagia and dysarthria.

2. Lesions of the pons often involve cranial nerves V, VII, and VIII. Facial paralysis, which could be nuclear in distribution, and loss of sensation are observed.

3. Lesions of the midbrain frequently involve cranial nerves III, IV, and VI. At that level, a variety of specific ocular palsy syndromes are noted.

Many cranial nerve lesions present as ipsilateral deficits. With the contralateral sensory deficits described above, they generate the clinical condition of crossed neurologic signs. Early in the course of the stroke, during shock, and when the patient is relaxed, these findings might not be easy to elicit. Accordingly, electrodiagnosis can facilitate the evaluation of the patient, especially with lesions of cranial nerves V and VII. Auditory-evoked potential technology can facilitate the evaluation of cranial nerve VIII lesions.[11-17]

Pending neurologic return, once these lesions have been diagnosed, rehabilitation goals become conservative and limited to preserving what remains of the function of that cranial nerve. Alternatively, the patient should be educated to perform whatever substitutions would aid function.[17-23] Medullary lesions produce the most dangerous lesions, as the dysphagia produced at times generates gram-negative aspiration pneumonia. The pneumonia can be recurrent, difficult to treat, and life threatening. Percutaneous gastrostomy techniques have helped treat this condition. However, this technique has now been performed so often in inpatients with hemorrhagic strokes that it threatens to become a substitute for adequate swallow therapy.

STRENGTH AND TONE

If the hemorrhagic stroke is large and widespread, the patient can present with deep, closed-eye coma and decerebrate rigidity. The muscles are rigid, and the limbs are held in extension. Much of the time, however, the extent of the hemorrhage into the brain stem will be limited or lacunar-like. This type of patient often presents with hemiparesis or even monoparesis rather than hemiplegia or monoplegia.[18-22,25] The intensity of the paralysis compares well in most cases with the intensity of the sensory deficit. These patients still have increased muscular tone and plastic rigidity, which limit precise muscular control and limb placement. Most of the time, patterned limb motion is still observed. But this patterned movement capacity can be used to restore function to most patients in feeding, grooming, bed mobility, and transfer activities. Patients so involved have been able to reach on occasion the functional level of modified independence for these activities.

Just as a patient with a hemorrhagic stroke of the posterior circulation could have intact function of the cerebral hemispheres, the patient could present with extensive sensory and motor deficits and yet retain active thought processes. At the extreme of the clinical spectrum, a "locked-in" syndrome can be generated. These locked-in patients are often affectively challenged. These people have feelings that they cannot fully express. Consequently, these patients' frustration, anxiety, depression, and anger can be intense. Much of the time, neurologic functional return is great enough to alleviate this stressful psychological situation.[11-19,25] Even under better circumstances, however, the patient could experience a major depression. In that circumstance, it could be difficult to determine if the patient has also acquired a significant cognitive deficit.

EFFECT ON REHABILITATION

Cranial nerves perform functions that are vital toward how patients sense and relate to the external world. They are "end nerves" in that generally their strategic and vital functions cannot be substituted by applying functions of another nerve. Small wonder that in these patients, the early post-ictal course is rough and turbulent, as these patients are blinded, at least temporarily, to the external environment, and the vital signs and neurologic status of these patients have not completely stabilized. In the rush to medically and neurologically stabilize these patients, rehabilitative concerns are frequently not top priority. Yet rehabilitation medicine is at optimal effectiveness if it is begun at this stage.

Aspiration pneumonia, deconditioning, decubitus ulcer generation, deep venous thrombosis, and indwelling catheter–related conditions are all complications commonly noted after admission of these patients to an acute inpatient rehabilitation ward. If the patient can be successfully managed through early stages, neurologic return usually facilitates an excellent functional recovery later in the medical course. The investment of adequate acute rehabilitation inpatient time is a key to this outcome.

At the beginning, nursing therapy demands are high, but corners should not be cut. Patience, careful care, and endless repetition are all important attributes for the rehabilitation team to express to these patients, their friends, and their families. Optimal functional return is consistently seen only after early and intensive rehabilitative care. These patients are often best treated when they remain on the rehabilitative ward despite acute complications and sequelae. Equipment required for communication or for activities of daily living should be received and used rapidly, seamlessly, and smoothly during rehabilitation. Later, those patients who do regain effective communication should be made to feel that they are an active part of the rehabilitation team. These people often feel that they have been inactive for too long, and they need to assert their personalities within the rehabilitation team process. They tend to become responsive to respect, friendship, and equality shown by the rehabilitation team. Patients who have progressed from a locked-in–type clinical condition and regained communication should be given the freedom, privacy, and space to express their feelings. They should be welcomed into the rehabilitation team even if that welcome also generates inconvenience or complications.

REFERENCES

1. Strich SJ. Diffuse degeneration of the cerebral white matter in severe dementia following head injury. *J Neurol Neurosurg Psychiatry* 1956;19:163.

2. Kakulas BA. The applied neuropathology of human spinal cord injury. *Spinal Cord* 1999;37:79–88.
3. Kakulas BA. A review of the neuropathology of human spinal cord injury with emphasis on special features. *J Spinal Cord Med* 1999;22:119–124.
4. Denny-Brown D, Russell WR. Experimental cerebral concussion. *Brain* 1941;64:93–164.
5. Whyte J, Rosenthal M. Rehabilitation of the patient with traumatic brain injury. In: DeLisa JA (ed). *Rehabilitation Medicine: Principles and Practice, second edition*. Philadelphia: Lippincott, 1993;825–860.
6. Maxwell WL, et al. A mechanistic analysis of nondisruptive axonal injury. *J Neurotrauma* 1997;14:419–440.
7. Brown WF, Boulton CF. *Clinical Electromyography*. Boston: Butterworth, 1984.
8. Kaplan PE, Tanner ED. *Musculoskeletal Pain and Disability*. Norwalk: Appleton & Lange, 1989.
9. Fisher CM, et al. Lateral medullary infarction. *J Neuropathol Exp Neurol* 1961;20:323–333.
10. Meythaler JM, et al. Current concepts: diffuse axonal injury-associated traumatic brain injury. *Arch Phys Med Rehabil* 2001; 82:1461–1471.
11. Adams R. Occlusion of the anterior inferior cerebellar artery. *Arch Neurol* 1943;49:765–771.
12. Amerenco P, Hauw JJ. Cerebellar infarction in the territory of the superior cerebellar artery. *Neurology* 1990;40:1383–1390.
13. Amerenco P, et al. Les infarctus du territoire de L'artere cerebelleuse posteroinferieure. *Rev Neurol* 1989;145:277–279.
14. Amerenco P, et al. Anterior inferior cerebellar artery territory infarcts. *Arch Neurol* 1993;50:154–161.
15. Barth A, Bogousslavsky J, Regli F. The clinical and topographic spectrum of cerebellar infarcts. *Ann Neurol* 1993;33:451–456.
16. Besson G, et al. Failure of magnetic resonance imaging in the detection of pontine lacune. *Stroke* 1992;23:153–155.
17. Bronstein AM. The visual vertigo syndrome. *Acta Otolaryngol* 1995;52 Suppl (OPtl):45–48.
18. Caplan LR. "Top of the basilar" syndrome. *Neurology* 1980;30:72–79.
19. Caplan LR. *Stroke: A Clinical Approach*. Boston: Butterworths, 1993.
20. Fisher CM, Karnes W, Kubik C. Lateral medullary infarction. *J Neuropathol Exp Neurol* 1961;20:323–333.
21. Glass JD, Levey Al, Rothstein JD. The dysarthria-clumsy hand syndrome. *Ann Neurol* 1990;27:487–494.
22. Goodhart SP, Davison C. Syndrome of the posterior inferior and anterior inferior cerebellar arteries and their branches. *Arch Neurol Psychiatry* 1936; 35:501–524.
23. Hommel M, Bogousslavsky J. The spectrum of vertical gaze palsy following unilateral brain stem stroke. *Neurology* 1991;41:1229–1234.
24. Kalita J, Misra UK. Motor and sensory evoked potential studies in brainstem stroke. *EMG Clin Neurophysiol* 1997;37:379–383.
25. Kaplan PE, Cerullo U. *Stroke Rehabilitation*. Boston: Butterworths, 1986.
26. Kubik C, Adams RD. Occlusion of the basilar artery. *Brain* 1946;69:73–121.
27. Lopez LI, et al. Clinical and MRI correlation in 27 patients with acquired pendular nystagmus. *Brain* 1996;119:465–72.

B

Organization of the Acute Rehabilitation Service

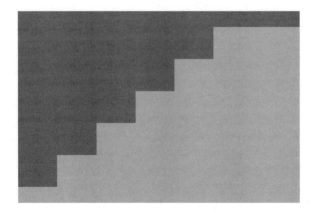

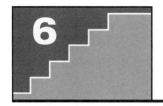

Influence of Premorbid Lifestyle

Paul E. Kaplan

This second group of chapters assumes that evaluation, differential diagnosis, and medical or surgical stabilization of the hemorrhagic stroke patient have all been completed. Consequently, guidance concerning the most effective medical, procedural, and surgical options that are curative for any specific complication of these patients is not emphasized. Hemorrhagic stroke disorders can, however, be managed, mitigated, and alleviated. Function can be restored, and self-sufficiency can be regained. This chapter focuses on the completion of a record of positive and negative contributing factors—factors that themselves add to or subtract from the cumulative rehabilitative medicine stress or strain and in that way increase or decrease the chances of an adverse rehabilitation outcome.

Risk factors have usually been associated with epidemiologic studies and include genetic, environmental, and medical factors that augment the risk of patients acquiring a stroke disorder.[1] The influence of genetic factors has been discussed in Chapter 2. Medical and genetic factors not only lead these patients to acquire their first strokes, but also lead these strokes to expand and for these patients to acquire new strokes during rehabilitation.[2] There is a strong direct association between hypertension and intracerebral hemorrhage.[3] Hypertension, however, also indirectly contributes to the acceleration of atherosclerosis.[4] As a result, hypertension also contributes as a risk factor to the chances of a population having an increased chance of acquiring thrombotic stroke.[5]

RISK FACTORS

Increased Strain on a Weakened System

Felix Mendelsohn, the composer, died at the age of 38 years after a hemorrhagic stroke that might have resulted from a ruptured aneurysm. An active, productive man, he had been under great stress from his duties in Leipzig and also from a newer job at the imperial court in Berlin. With Mendelsohn, the results probably were due to increased stress having been applied to a weakened organ system.

Although the overall reported incidence of hemorrhagic stroke declined during the 1960s and 1970s, it has leveled off[6–24] and has even demonstrated during this decade a resurgence, with increased prevalence, morbidity, and mortality.[6–13,20–24] Lifestyles involving high physical stress levels are associated with increased morbidity and mortality due to hemorrhagic stroke. Stress promotes the onset of stroke syndromes (ictus) through the generation of musculoskeletal failure and muscular exhaustion. Musculoskeletal failure itself is manifested through pain, stiffness, weakness, and numbness. Consequently, patients with musculoskeletal failure expend more energy and effort to perform the same set of functional actions than they might have had to expend if musculoskeletal failure had not occurred.[11–15] With added exertion, blood pressure rises, increasing the risk for hemorrhagic stroke onsets and ictus.

Failure of function within the musculoskeletal system is generally not spontaneous. It occurs within a specific context often elicited within the initial history. The patient often lists these situations spontaneously during the telling of his or her story. Musculoskeletal failure then augments the quality and quantity of physical stress in an open feedback loop. The stress-failure cycle formed after the application of stress can alter the normal function of both hormonal and immune body mechanisms (Figure 6.1).

The stress-failure cycle within each patient increases signs and symptoms of pain, tenderness, stiffness, and weakness and numbness. Therefore, after musculoskeletal failure, specific clinical patterns can be frequently observed that in themselves demonstrate specific signs and symptoms.

The following three special conditions are associated with musculoskeletal failure:

1. *Normal stress or strain has been applied to a weakened musculoskeletal system.* A normal person has been weakened through a musculoskeletal injury and then subjected to normal stress. An example is the basketball player who strains his right arm during work at home and then later goes for a lay-up during a basketball game.

2. *Augmented stress or strain has been applied to a normal musculoskeletal system.* A normal person has been suddenly subjected to increased stress. An example is the hockey player who experiences a vigorous and unexpected body check during a hockey game.

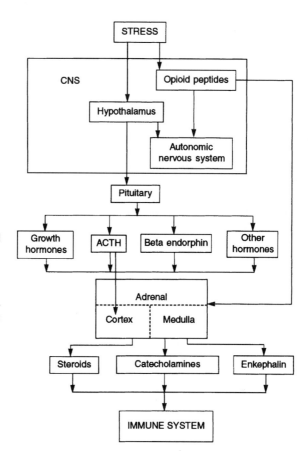

Figure 6.1 Applied stress, modifying the function of both hormonal and immune systems. (ACTH = adrenocorticotropic hormone; CNS = central nervous system.) (Reprinted with permission from Cailliet R. *Pain: Mechanisms and Management.* Philadelphia: F.A. Davis, 1993.)

3. *Augmented stress or strain has been applied to an already weakened musculoskeletal system.* A normal person with a weakened musculoskeletal system is then subjected to increased stress. An example is the patient who has just spent all weekend moving heavy pieces of furniture at home and is asked at work Monday morning to lift a heavy piece of equipment. This type of condition is most often noted when taking the histories of patients who have had hemorrhagic strokes.

As an added complication, augmented stress itself, over time, primarily modifies musculoskeletal structure and function. It also weakens the media wall layer of small-caliber arterioles within the central nervous system. Normally elastic and resilient, these arterioles become more brittle and fragile under the full weight of hypertension and increased cardiac work. The neurovascular supply of oxygen to the central nervous system has been diminished. The full destructive effect of hemorrhagic stroke on the central nervous system is therefore increased because of the application of augmented strain applied to the already weakened defenses of the central nervous system.[3-18] Because the application of elevated physical stress on a weakened musculoskeletal system produces hemorrhagic stroke, reducing that physical stress level helps prevent hemorrhagic strokes.

The results are apparent when taking a history from these patients. These patients consistently reveal premorbid lifestyles replete with negative and self-destructive impulses. The full manifestation of this lifestyle could vary. However, the particulars will have been expressed in some fashion by these patients and their companions over a period of years, even decades. This particular type of history has rendered these patients "geriatric" during their young adult and middle-aged adult years. Many of these patients also have college or professional degrees or hold positions in the business world of middle-level executives but are not working anywhere near optimal levels.

Addictive Behavior and Medication

Addictive behavior is frequently found in patients at risk for hemorrhagic stroke and their close families and companions. It places these patients at a much higher risk for hemorrhagic stroke.[6-17] The regular, frequent use of prescription medication generates similar problems. In both situations, being relaxed is an internal emotional condition that is responsive to a specific external stimulus. Inner tension or anxiety cannot be treated for a long time by these external means. Moreover, increasing needs for higher doses of medication to obtain the initial medication effect itself generates an ever-expanding demand for more of the applied substance. Internal emotional stress levels lead to the accelerated intake of chemicals that produce elevated physical stress levels. Although affective or mood stress has been muted, the cost is augmented physical stress. The overall physical stress levels might not have originally been moderate, but after the ingestion of addictive substances or medication, physical stress levels can be high.

One of the main categories of substances used is stimulants, especially caffeine, nicotine, and stimulant medications. Anabolic steroids and their performance-enhancing variants have diverse, complex effects, but the overall effect on the body is not noticeably different from those medications in the stimulant category. These all also produce tachycardia and increase cardiac output and hypertension episodically. During these episodes, effectiveness of the neurovascular blood supply is reduced.[14-21] This combination places maximum pressure on and within smaller caliber arterioles of the central nervous system. Subsequent relaxation does not reduce the immediate strain generated by these type of medications. Over time, these medications augment contractile periods by arteriolar wall musculature, the rate of smooth muscle proliferation in vessel walls, the rate of destruction at the cellular level of the intima of these blood vessels, and the rate of atherosclerotic deterioration of the wall of the blood vessel. This natural evolution has the effect of subjecting innate deficits, strains, and fissures within the musculature of the blood vessels of the central nervous system to stress that enhances these deficits.[6–8,12,14–18]

This type of clinical course started by stimulants can also be seen with those people who have been placed on antidepressant medication, especially tricyclic medication, monoamine oxidase inhibitors, and dextroamphetamine and related medication. For example, although the process of the generation of the muscular defect that yields an intracerebral aneurysm remains a mystery, this type of acquired stress imposed over decades definitely would not slow the aneurysm generation process down and might contribute to the size or depth of that defect. Superimposed changes in the wall of the surrounding tissue would only accelerate the changes in the wall of the involved blood vessel and contribute to the hemorrhagic stroke (Figure 6.2).

Another chemical category consists of major and minor depressants. Among the major depressants are antiseizure, antipsychotic, hypnotic, sedative, and opiate medications. Among the other substances are many recreational medications, alcohol, and tranquilizer medications.

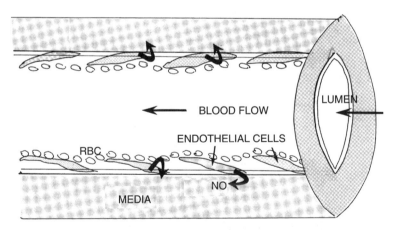

Figure 6.2 Shear stress on endothelial cells: control of arterial lumen. Blood flow that increases from exercise and elevated heartbeat causes an increase in peripheral blood flow from increase in arterial lumen. This would appear contradictory, as compression of the vessels from active peripheral muscles should decrease the lumen. As the blood flow increases, the deformed endothelial cells secrete a substance similar to nitric oxide (NO), which intrinsically relaxes the medial fibers and increases the lumen. (RBC = red blood cells.)

Contrast temperature baths once were applied to atherosclerotic or vasculitis conditions of the lower limbs. They have fallen into disuse because these baths have, in some specific cases, accelerated progress of the vasculitis. Depressants have had similar physiologic results. When blood levels of depressants rise, both bradycardia and relative hypotension ensue. Typically, however, when blood levels of these medications start to decline, the patient experiences a compensatory episodic tachycardia and hypertension. Neurovascular central nervous system tone will have been accented. Many patients progress to constantly reactive tachycardia and hypertension.[12–21] However, the usual biphasic response alone is quite great enough to significantly stress the central nervous system.

Analgetic and antihistamine medications—and especially nonsteroidal anti-inflammatory drugs (NSAIDs)—often demonstrate the same biphasic response noted above with depressant medications. Furthermore, when combined with stimulant medication, significant elevations of cardiac output, pulse, blood pressure, and cardiac work are frequently observed. Some NSAIDs share similar mechanisms and enzymes with antidepressant medications modifying serotonin metabolism. Accordingly, conditions have been set promoting hemorrhagic stroke. What was a small defect in a small-caliber artery with time becomes a vessel with a leak. Eventually, full rupture, subarachnoid hemorrhage, and ictus may be observed. This progression is driven by the patient taking one or more of these medications.[13–21] Many patients are intense, competitive, and have little insight into their dependency on medication. Denial is a common emotional defense. Reliance on combination medication and medication taken with alcoholic beverages is a very common additive risk factor.

Natural food supplements can act within the same methods, but these medications have even less federal regulation. Kava root, for example, usually acts as a minor depressant. St. John's wort usually acts as a stimulant. When combined with other substances, these compounds can contribute to the results described above. These effects are in addition to side effects that include arthralgia, myalgia, weakness, and pain. Natural food supplements can generate all of the complications and sequelae seen in prescription medications. It is important, therefore, that the history taken from young and middle-aged adults go into both psychological and physical habits and addictions. The interaction of prescription stimulant medications, coffee intake, and smoking is poorly understood, but nicotine and caffeine are both stimulants and might well facilitate stimulant effects of prescription medications. It is thought that smoking cigarettes does potentiate subarachnoid hemorrhage and also the complication of delayed cerebral ischemia. Recreational medications that are stimulants have the same potential.

Excessive Physical and Emotional Stress

One accepted method of treating internal stress is by excessive physical exercise. Alone, heavy aerobic exercises might well promote optimal body conditioning. Endorphin production certainly leads to feelings of well-being. When dietary fads and fashions are added, this new combination changes the clinical situation. Under these new circumstances, these types of exercise programs (e.g., marathon running and lifting weights) increase cardiac output, pulse, blood pressure, and cardiac work in exhausted athletes.[17-24] Inappropriate, exaggerated therapeutic exercise and dietary programs punish the body through increasing physical stress.

Some diets are often unbalanced and amount to starvation. A clinical situation, therefore, has been created during which increased stress has been placed on a weakened system. For example, a long-distance speed bike rider comes home after a 75-mile course and collapses with a ruptured aneurysm. Is this really a coincidence, or has an internal deficit been magnified by tremendously high self-imposed physical stress levels? Serial coronary angiograms show that patients with angina and stenosed coronary arteries have completely occluded one or more of these coronary arteries during the time that they have augmented their exercise tolerances. Is this truly cardiac rehabilitation?

Being under great emotional duress is thought to be the equivalent of ascending three flights of stairs. Whether the stress has been physical or emotional, cardiac output, pulse, blood pressure, and cardiac work have all been increased. If the patient has been emotionally disturbed over time, the same pattern of physical strain and food deprivation is often observed. Chances are that the patient will be a smoker. The problem is that leakage from an aneurysm or from pinpoint hemorrhagic strokes into the cerebral hemispheres produces a picture of exhaustion, headache, and fatigue that will be thought part of the physical or emotional stress.[15-18] Two other dietary patterns—binge/purge and anorexia—also place an unwelcome stress on the central nervous system.

Two additional sources of stress are obesity and spasticity.[10-15] They are both aversive factors to rehabilitation management. Obesity usually reduces available coordination capacity, makes transfer activities difficult for the team and patient, increases the risk of falling, prolongs the wound healing from any surgical procedure, and increases the risk of complications and sequelae. Spasticity, at times caused from previous strokes, uses abnormal muscular control to increase the metabolic cost of even the simplest motor activity such as during feeding activities. The origin of spasticity—and its augmented metabolic costs—is associated with hyperactive spinal stretch reflexes (Figure 6.3).

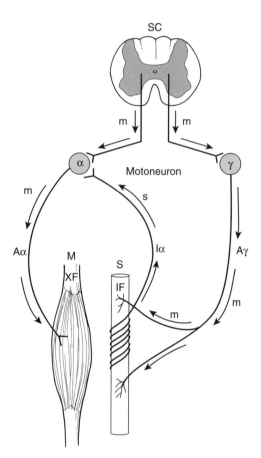

Figure 6.3 Spinal stretch reflex: supra-spinal influence. The extrafusal fibers (XF) of the skeletal muscle (M) and the intrafusal fibers (IF) of the spindle system (S) are innervated by the motoneurons alpha (α) and gamma (γ). These fibers descend from the spinal cord (SC). The motor fibers (m) motorize the muscle fibers via A alpha (Aα) fibers. The spindle system is sensory (s) back to the cord via the I alpha (Iα) fibers. The spindle system is "reset" by the motoneuron γ fibers via A gamma (Aγ) fibers. (Modified from Zimmerman M. Regulatory functions of the nervous system, as exemplified by the spinal motor system. In Schmidt RF [ed], *Fundamentals of Neurophysiology*. New York: Springer-Verlag, 1985.)

Prognostic Effect

The two most consistent risk factors for hemorrhagic stroke are high cardiac output and high cardiac work. They are commonly high because of hypertensive heart disease that is not adequately managed due either to noncompliance or to substandard therapy.[7–11] Although consistently augmented daily blood pressures are harmful, it is usually the enormously high episodic peaks of hypertension that are frequently implicated.

Other risk factors that are harmful but not as much as these special hypertensive episodes are blood dyscrasia and any medical condition or drug that would unusually dilate arterioles of the central nervous system, as seen in many of the treatments for migraine headaches. Another condition that has many of these features is pregnancy, or, alternatively, many of the complications noted when taking birth control medication. With most patients, these risk factors are easy to find. Indeed, combinations of these risk factors are frequent when these patients and their families are studied, usually after the fact. These patients represent in a real sense the casualties of the stress built into modern life and culture. It would be difficult in any one patient to prove that anything has significantly changed the absolute rate at which intrinsic deficits lead to newly acquired intracranial aneurysms. It is much more effective to alter preventive stress-related factors that help generate hemorrhagic stroke.

POSITIVE CONTRIBUTING FACTORS AIDING IN RECOVERY FROM HEMORRHAGIC STROKE

Just as certain risk factors help generate a hemorrhagic stroke, certain positive factors aid in functional recovery after a hemorrhagic stroke. When two or more of these positive conditions are present, it makes the efforts of the rehabilitation team that much more effective and efficient. These helpful, friendly, positive factors make it much easier to help the patient become an active, participating member of the rehabilitation team.

When these patients are a part of the team, they are aided in their efforts by the knowledge that even though they have been injured, they have done their best to respond and to adapt. As functional return is not necessarily dependent on neurologic return, a patient could still have experienced a relatively serious hemorrhagic stroke with little neurologic return, as a worst case example, and still could have the chance of becoming functionally independent or functionally independent with the use of appropriate equipment. Generally, however, hemorrhagic stroke is intrinsically different from thrombotic stroke. Hemorrhagic stroke generally has greater neurologic return than thrombotic stroke, but also greater chances of repeat ictal events. With each patient, however, the chances of functional return after a hemorrhagic stroke are significantly aided by the increased possibilities of neurologic recovery.

Degree of Physical Conditioning

After strokes and after spinal cord injuries, it has been noted in several studies that patients who have been athletes become medically stable sooner and have fewer complications. But not all athletic builds are alike. Generally, athletes that are tough, thin, agile, and not too heavy or tall do better.

Weight can be a problem—even if the majority of that weight is muscle—because it will make that patient just a little less agile. Coordination, both gross and fine motor, is much more important than strength for mobility activities and also for activities of daily living. On the other hand, the combination of deconditioning and excessive weight generates complications and sequelae for that slow-to-heal patient. Athletic conditioning programs are also not really equivalent. Weight lifting usually does not produce the agility that water sports generate. There is great variation in the expression of this positive factor.

Amount of Neurologic and Functional Recovery

The amount of natural neurologic and functional recovery after a stroke has been noted through the years based on thousands of clinical observations. This classic model, based on what Francis Bacon called *nature's own laboratory*, is a learning-curve–type clinical evolution through time. The evolution can plateau at any stage, thus affecting the amount of the patient's eventual clinical functional recovery. Therefore, for example, the onset of spasticity is an unfavorable risk factor, as the amount of possible functional return decreases by 25% (Figure 6.4).

Data correlated using neurologic assessment, functional assessment, and magnetic resonance imaging examinations lead to different conclusions. In fact, the estimated neurologic and functional recoveries after a hemorrhagic stroke are significantly more optimistic than those after a thrombotic stroke.[21–24] The classic model described above includes both types of stroke. Patients after hemorrhagic stroke usually respond faster and more completely to physical rehabilitation than expected in the classic model, especially if rehabilitation is begun early after ictus. The actual natural history of a hemorrhagic stroke is not necessarily a continuous, straight line–type of process. It can stop and start again. Complications and sequelae provide detours. There is no real deadline. No time duration after ictus will eliminate the chance of and opportunity for significant neurologic and functional recoveries. Spasticity can appear and then disappear during the application of therapeutic exercises after ictus. In its turn, the hope of neurologic and functional recoveries motivates the patient and his or her family to do better.

Degree of Emotional and Mental Flexibility

The ability to reformulate attitudes while under stressful conditions is at the heart of the rehabilitative process. This ability is universal and innate but commonly not cultivated. As these central nervous system injuries are both unexpected and unforeseen, this flexibility is a strate-

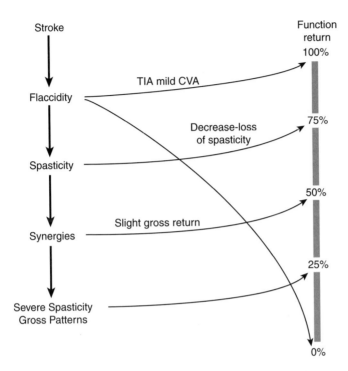

Stroke

Flaccidity

TIA mild CVA

Spasticity

Decrease-loss
of spasticity

Synergies

Slight gross return

Severe Spasticity
Gross Patterns

Function
return
100%

75%

50%

25%

0%

Figure 6.4 The classic model of estimated functional recovery after a stroke. (CVA = cerebrovascular accident; TIA = transient ischemic attack.) (Reprinted with permission from Cailliet R. *Shoulder in Hemiplegia*. Philadelphia: F.A. Davis, 1980.)

gic factor. This specific ability involves a more active approach rather than passively keeping an open mind, as it also includes the combination of being innovative, realistic, and creative.

The flexibility should be present in friends and family as well as in the patient. To become members of the rehabilitative team, these patients, their friends, and their family should be able to view positive aspects of their situation and therefore be qualified to use these positive aspects to further their abilities. Many advances in rehabilitative care have been generated within this context. If the patient and his or her circle of extended family is therefore positive, helpful, and friendly, the rehabilitative team functions more effectively and efficiently, producing greater functional outcome with lower costs.

Ability to Invent and Improvise

The rehabilitative team usually tries to customize the rehabilitative program to each patient and not to a specific diagnosis. This factor is usually associated closely with the team's degree of emotional and cognitive flexibility. The goal of the rehabilitation team in this factor is to make the most efficient and effective use of the material at hand to solve functional problems. Rehabilitative patients clever enough with materials provided to address specific functional difficulties can provide the instigation for these types of solutions. It is only through practical innovation and pragmatism that the rehabilitative patient, friends, and family become active participants in the rehabilitative team.

If positive attitudes initiate the rehabilitative team process, performing daily, realistic, and practical jobs help sustain that process. The patient, friends, and family must risk daily failure, pain, and weakness to build a new and relevant infrastructure to the patient's daily life activities so that life is meaningful. Acute rehabilitation inpatient wards in this way become environments that foster rapid change and therefore produce greater rates of functional improvement through time. During the rehabilitation process, the patient is encouraged to be adaptive, flexible, opportunistic, and, especially, assertive.

Support from Family and Friends

A large, loving, supportive family or extended family involved with the patient's care can shorten the rehabilitation stay and profoundly change the nature of the subsequent disposition. Health maintenance organization–type rehabilitative programs that actually encourage early outpatient care rely on this factor. It can be overrated.

One of the really difficult moments in a rehabilitative stay comes toward the end. At that point, family and friends are enlisted to spend actual time, effort, and energy to help sustain the rehabilitative momentum that the patient has created and maintained through the inpatient hospital stay. Committing to a daily grind of mobility and self-care activities and then remaining reliable is not glamorous. Recruiting the effort needed is not easy.

When, and if, an extended family does sign up for a patient care program and follow-up with home therapeutic visits to meet specific rehabilitation goals, the patient is strengthened, supported, and given a better opportunity to achieve success. When a patient is surrounded by a supportive extended family, community re-entry is also more successful. This factor can open a wide variety of pre-vocational and vocational opportunities in his or her home community.

EFFECT ON REHABILITATION

Preventive rehabilitation is the most effective and efficient type of rehabilitation medicine. Alteration of lifestyle can repeatedly prevent or decrease the full effects of hemorrhagic stroke. For example, patients who are in good physical condition at ictus have a much better outcome functionally than those who are overweight and deconditioned. However, it is not common to receive patients in good to excellent physical condition. Contributing factors in prevention include hypertension control, stress reduction, and preservation of the neurovascular blood supply to the central nervous system, which is responsive to even small deficits in its oxygen supply for even brief intervals, by reduction of alcohol and recreational drug intake and smoking. Of these contributing factors, programs to control hypertension, reduce inner stress and strains, and promote physical conditioning can be especially effective in promoting the benefits of the therapy provided by the team to the patient. Stress reduction and conditioning programs can also help build and maintain a rehabilitation team's efficiency in the face of the burdens of patients who are more medically complex and demanding. Effective stress reduction and physical conditioning are effective preventive rehabilitation. Effective preventive rehabilitation can lengthen both the amount of life and the quality of life for each patient. Prevention also reduces the costs of medical care for that patient and also for society.

REFERENCES

1. Folger WN. Epidemiology of cerebrovascular disease. In Brandstater ME, Basmajian JV (eds). *Stroke Rehabilitation*. Baltimore: Williams & Wilkins, 1987;1–35.
2. Baker RN, *et al*. Prognosis among survivors of ischemic stroke. *Neurology* 1968;18:933–941.
3. Veterans Administration Cooperative Study Group on Antihypertensive Agents. Effects of treatment on morbidity in hypertension: Results in patients with diastolic blood pressure averaging 115 through 129 mm Hg. *JAMA* 1967;202:1028–1034.
4. Baker AB, *et al*. Hypertension and cerebral atherosclerosis. *Circulation* 1969;39:701–710.
5. Kannel WB, *et al*. Components of blood pressure and risk of atherothrombotic brain infarction: The Framingham Study. *Stroke* 1976;7:327–331.
6. Alter M, *et al*. Cerebrovascular disease: Frequency and population selectivity in an upper midwestern community. *Stroke* 1970;1:454–465.
7. Bamford J, *et al*. A prospective study of cerebrovascular disease in the community: The Oxfordshire Community Stroke Project 1981–86. Methodology, demography and incident cases of first-ever stroke. *J Neurol Neurosurg Psychiatry* 1988;51:1373–1380.
8. Barnett HJM. Prevention of stroke. *Am J Med* 1980;69:803–806.
9. Berlowitz DF, *et al*. Inadequate management of blood pressure in a hypertensive population. *N Engl J Med* 1998;339:1957–1963.

10. Broderick JP, *et al.* Incidence rates of stroke in the eighties: The end of the decline in stroke? *Stroke* 1989;20:577–582.
11. Carolei A, *et al.* High incidence in the prospective community-based L'Aquila registry (1994–1998). *Stroke* 1997;28:2500–2506.
12. Furlan AJ, Whisnant JP, Elveback LR. The decreasing incidence of primary intracerebral hemorrhage: A population study. *Ann Neurol* 1979;5:367–373.
13. Heyman A, *et al.* Cerebrovascular disease in the biracial population of Evans County, Georgia. *Stroke* 1971;2:509–518.
14. Kagan A, Popper JS, Rhoads GG. Factors related to stroke incidence in Hawaii Japanese men: The Honolulu Heart Study. *Stroke* 1980;11:14–21.
15. Kannel WB, *et al.* Systolic blood pressure, arterial rigidity, and the risk of stroke: The Framingham Study. *JAMA* 1981;245:1225–1229.
16. Kaplan CP, Corrigan JD. Effect of blood alcohol level on recovery from severe closed head injury. *Brain Injury* 1992;6:337–349.
17. Kaplan PE, Cerullo LJ. *Stroke Rehabilitation.* Boston: Butterworths, 1986.
18. Ostfeld AM, *et al.* Epidemiology of stroke in an elderly welfare population. *Am J Pub Health* 1974;64:450–458.
19. Phillips L, *et al.* The unchanging pattern of subarachnoid hemorrhage in a community. *Neurology* 1980;30:1034–1040.
20. Royal College of Physicians. Disability and rehabilitation. Report by the Royal College of Physicians. London, 1993.
21. Sorensen PS, *et al.* Prevalence of stroke in a district of Copenhagen. *Acta Neurol Scand* 1982;66:68–81.
22. Veterans Administration Cooperative Study Group on Antihypertensive Agents. Effects of treatment on morbidity in hypertension. 11 Results in patients with diastolic blood pressure averaging 90 through 114 mm Hg. *JAMA* 1970;213:1143–1152.
23. Wolf PA. An overview of the epidemiology of stroke. *Stroke* 1990;21(Suppl 11):11–46.
24. Yekutiel M, *et al.* The prevalence of hypertension, ischemia heart disease and diabetes in traumatic spinal cord injured patients and amputees. *Paraplegia* 1989;27:58–62.

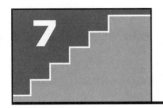

Deficits of Function to be Addressed

Paul E. Kaplan

Physical burdens make the rehabilitation of the stroke patient more difficult. The two physical burdens that the rehabilitation team have to control and reduce are pain and weakness, and of these two physical obstructions to progress, pain is the most urgent. Strengthening exercises are effective after the challenge of pain has been managed. Research performed during the investigation of mechanical hyperalgesia has helped to reveal a complex and relevant neurophysiologic infrastructure. In fact, peripheral nervous system inputs to the central nervous system can generate enhanced responses, or central sensitization.[1] Examples of an enhanced response include light tactile stimuli, producing pain (e.g., dynamic hyperalgesia) in patients with reflex sympathetic dystrophy or thalamic strokes.[2,3] Another type of hyperalgesia also seen in stroke patients is static hyperalgesia, and this hyperalgesia is generated by pin-prick stimulations.[4-6] Whereas static hyperalgesia is usually associated with inputs of mechano-sensitive nociceptors, dynamic hyperalgesia is associated with the inputs of low-threshold mechanoreceptors.[1,7,8] After cutaneous injuries, dynamic hyperalgesia can be managed much more easily than static hyperalgesia.[9,10] These studies suggest that within the right type of environment—stroked, not punctate—central nervous system sensitization may be controlled and modified. However, much more remains to be done in the study of the generation of pain. The pattern of progress within rehabilitation management is that certain empirically generated methodologies are effective and are then investigated by subsequent scientific clinical and basic research. This chapter presents some of these principles and their subsequent applications toward medical rehabilitative therapy.[11-25] The following principles and their applications produce much of the milieu in which the rehabilitation medicine team is built, is maintained, and works.

1. The process of rehabilitation is complex, involving relevant areas of legal, social, economic, and educational importance.

2. Relevant issues are vital to the formation and maintenance of the rehabilitation team through time. Team unity, harmony, and communication are most important.

3. The rehabilitation team commonly includes, but is not limited to, physicians, nurses, occupational therapists, physical therapists, speech pathologists, social workers, psychologists, vocational rehabilitation counselors, and recreational therapy counselors. The team, therefore, represents diverse educational levels, cultures, and disciplines, and goodwill will need to be built.

DOES FUNCTIONAL RETURN DEPEND ON THE DEGREE OF NEUROLOGIC RETURN?

The quantitative amount of functional return and the qualitative lifestyle status are only partially dependent on neurologic return. Should the patient experience a significant neurologic return during the rehabilitative care process, the patient will have a much better chance of experiencing true self-sufficiency by the end of that process. If the patient has experienced rehabilitative therapy and then experiences neurologic return, the quality and quantity of his or her functional return are aided. Should the patient, however, develop such complications and sequelae as contractures, severe deconditioning, or decubitus ulcers, the patient would probably not realize his or her full rehabilitation potential, even if the patient subsequently experiences neurologic return. Legal implications, however, are ever present, and the onset of any of the complications or sequelae named above could be considered part of the error of practice.

Two examples illustrate the daily reality of this type of medical care.

1. A patient with hemorrhagic stroke of the dominant middle cerebral artery territory and global aphasia can be taught nonverbal methods of self-care even if the global aphasia only evolves to a dense receptive aphasia.[11–13,17] In fact, teaching activities of daily living to a nonverbal patient with global aphasia is often less difficult than teaching those tasks to a patient with dense receptive aphasia. If those patients can be taught to transfer and to groom themselves, they then require much less care and are easier to place with a relative or friend. Should neurologic return then occur, these patients are that much more likely to become fully functionally independent.

2. A patient with stroke hemorrhages into the territory of the anterior cerebral arteries bilaterally and experiences cerebral paraplegia. If

this patient's sensation deficits and bilateral leg, ankle, and foot weaknesses remain unchanged, orthoses can be provided as well as intensive gait and transfer therapy. With adequate treatment on the ward and follow-up after discharge, safe limited ambulation may be achieved.[14,16,20] The patient needs to be able to respond to sensory retraining techniques. If neurologic return occurred, therapy would be made much easier and much more effective. The partial contributions of rehabilitative team therapy and neurologic return toward full patient self-sufficiency in his or her community generate the following significant corollaries:

a. Rehabilitative therapy tends to produce patients who are more emotionally stable, mentally adaptable, and physically fit. Those patients will be better able to use their musculoskeletal system.

b. Rehabilitative functional progress is frequently not an equal, steady, or orderly progression toward self-sufficiency. Progress is irregular and is monitored by functional outcome scales.

c. The progress of rehabilitation is most often slow at the beginning and slows again toward the end of the rehabilitation stay.

d. Activities of daily living, housekeeping, transfer activities, wheelchair/standing/gait activities, equipment needs, communication needs, and socialization needs are usually included.

Even under optimal circumstances, broadly based progress in all of these areas is usually uneven and lower than expectations, barring neurologic return.[11-16] There are well over 50 functional outcome scales in regular national use today. Many scales are digital, computer friendly, national, and broadly applied. Some scales are specific to a few diseases or disorders.

The majority of functional outcome scales consist of equivalent intervals, even though functional progress does not usually resemble that model.[15,18,21-24] Ordinal intervals could be transformed to resemble the nonequivalent data of most rehabilitative processes. Equivalent interval data itself can be analyzed using exponential statistical methodology. At least one national organization has encouraged this modification. Rehabilitative progress is unique and inimitable to each patient's situation and to each rehabilitation team's condition. The following should be kept in mind when measuring functional outcomes:

1. Whatever functional outcome system is used, the rehabilitation team should take into account patient safety, human error, and human variability.

2. Patient progress estimation should be accurate and realistic.

3. Are these patients or their families ready and able to participate in a rehabilitation program? Rehabilitation is an elective medical service.

4. Has effective, efficient communication been established between these patients/families and the rest of the rehabilitation team?

5. Is the rehabilitation team ready, willing, and able to accept this participation and communication, even though that participation consumes time and energy?

When functional outcome measurement began, one viewpoint applied a national standard (NS).[16–20] Those generally subscribing to this view have succeeded in generating functional outcome scales used on a national context. In the process, these scales have been used to limit the amount of funding for the rehabilitation of patients based essentially on a national data pool for each condition by establishing "windows" of cost-effective rehabilitation for each condition.

Difficulties with NS scales abound. If rehabilitation enhances hygiene and bed mobility and thus prevents decubitus ulcers, this rehabilitative process is worth funding even if it does not generate many units on NS functional outcome scales. The alternative viewpoint concerns itself with the practical goals of each inpatient rehabilitation team's effort. This relative standard (RS) was initially supported by the American Medical Association. Each devolved unit would contend for itself how much functional outcome could be generated for each unit of cost. This RS viewpoint contends that each rehabilitation team should monitor its goals in its own setting in an analogue, narrative manner during rehabilitation.[12–14] So far, health maintenance organization (HMO) funding for rehabilitation medicine clinical service has relied on the NS positions rather than those of RS. The rehabilitation process, however, must still be characterized. The following may be used to define rehabilitation progress:

1. Logical inconsistencies frequently trap many well-meaning attempts to fully characterize the rehabilitation medicine process.

2. Applying objective research methods to a process or entity that is basically subjective leads to misleading results. Much literature on chronic pain syndrome falls into this disadvantage. But NS methodology also contributes, as it applies national and regional objective, digital techniques to measuring a process that is relatively analogue or subjective.

3. Neurologic progress is not necessarily fully documented through serial magnetic resonance images. One way of addressing these types of debates regarding functional progress of inpatients is through the documentation of regular, serial neurologic and functional assessments.

Inpatients on an acute rehabilitation unit should be team evaluated in this way on at least a weekly basis. The team conference membership should consist of those therapists, nurses, and aides who are actually working with that particular patient. Substitutions should be kept rare and by prior agreement. Nonessential but interested bystanders should be discouraged from attending by the team facilitator, as confidentiality of these team proceedings is important. Videotaping or audiotaping of a rehabilitation team conference would generate the same concerns.

To build a team consensus and communication, these patients and their families might be brought in to participate during parts of the conference. Many times, the same goal can be achieved by separate family conferences. Too many conferences (e.g., admitting, discharge, and family) are commonly resented by the rehabilitation team.

Results, however, of the rehabilitation team consensus and communication should be documented. Narrative notes should be in place when or shortly after events occur in a readable, thorough, accurate manner. Because these notes are carefully examined by HMOs, wording of these notes to capture the spirit and the letter of the team interaction is vital. Notes taken during the meeting can be dictated later.

ARE ALL FUNCTIONAL DEFICITS EQUAL?

No, all functional deficits are not equal. For example, in managing a patient after a hemorrhagic stroke, bed mobility independence and grooming activity independence widens the placement opportunities available for that patient. This fact is true and relevant even if that patient does not regain the ability to functionally ambulate. Yet many patients and their families enter the rehabilitation process with the firm idea that gait independence is a vital part of rehabilitation and with the expectation that he or she will be able to independently ambulate by the end of the rehabilitation process. Patients, significant others, and family often resist education efforts by the team, even as they respond physically to training directions. Evaluating geriatric patients often poses special challenges.

1. Geriatric patients require special considerations, as they often have special needs.

2. Elderly patients with hemorrhagic strokes, especially if they also have adult-onset diabetes and peripheral vascular or nerve disease, frequently are not able to ambulate without help. That help could be equipment, orthoses, or human aid.

3. Geriatric patients have a higher risk of falling episodes, hip fractures, pulmonary embolism, and death. NS functional outcome scales

do have safety considerations incorporated, but not necessarily effectively or efficiently in the rating system.[19-25] Safety issues should be part of the narrative rehabilitation team summary for legal as well as medical imperatives.

If a narrative summary as described above is entered in the patient's chart, these safety issues will have been accurately documented. In this way, the weekly narrative summary is really an expression of the status of the rehabilitation contract between the patient, the patient's family, and the rehabilitation team. Some rehabilitation teams even have a written contract that is signed, especially for complex disorders with medicolegal aspects such as chronic pain syndrome management or for patients or families who are litigious.

Whether oral or written, the contract should state the expectations as well as specific obligations of the patient, the patient's family, and the rehabilitation team. Each party should have performance expectations clarified in so far as that is possible. The consequences of the failure of that performance also should be addressed at the start of the rehabilitation program.

The rehabilitation contract usually requires frequent revision, as rehabilitation is, after all, human. The contract commonly needs modification with deterioration of these patients' medical or neurologic stability. This deterioration could take place with any of the major complications noted in patients with hemorrhagic strokes (see Chapter 8).

Mistakes and failures are part of the learning curve for all of the contract participants. Each contract should be fashioned according to these patients' needs and to the local and focal therapeutic environment. Without a successfully negotiated, and re-negotiated, rehabilitation contract, the rehabilitation process will be significantly suboptimal.

MULTIDISCIPLINARY CONSIDERATIONS

Thus far, the rehabilitation team has been discussed largely as one unit. That heterogeneous team, however, is subject to internal stress as well as external demands. In fact, internal and external tensions and stress help maintain a destructive dialectic tension far into the team rehabilitation process. Augmenting this tendency in the United States are regionally oriented trends of rugged individualism that act to slow and impede incorporation of separate professionals representing different disciplines in the rehabilitation team process. Whether the team is to be democratic, representative, or autocratic is a local, focal, and political issue. A central role of the team facilitator is therefore that of a team mediator preventing the growth of real discontent. The positive, helpful, and friendly way to accomplish that goal is to encourage cooperation and collegiality within the team. The following are further suggestions for building the rehabilitation team:

1. Every therapist on the rehabilitation team deserves and should expect respect, and the team should gather and nurture harmony.
2. Each member of the team should listen and think, as well as speak.
3. Other members of the team have needs to be understood and negotiated in a context of beneficence and goodwill.
4. Remember that members of the team are trying to participate as fully as they can.

Shorter hospital stays mandated by insurance companies and HMOs mean that there is more stress on negotiated agreements within the rehabilitation team than there is time available to mediate that tension. In the past, inpatient stays were commonly extended until many of the equipment-related loose ends or threads had been tied. The patient was able to be discharged, equipment in hand, with home health services already organized and ready to begin.

Now, these patients and their families are frequently forced to rely on more rapidly organized efforts. As a result of the Balanced Budget Act of 1997, the financial basis of medical care of chronic diseases (e.g., rehabilitation medicine, cancer care, and psychiatric care) has been greatly reduced. The critical mass of therapists, clinicians, and nurses vital to the rehabilitation medicine process has been drastically limited. The mechanism for this type of reduction has been through the imposition of the artificial floor and glass ceiling as noted under Dealing with the Artificial Floor and Glass Ceiling. Financial support for both skilled nursing units and home health service management has been severely compromised. With uncomplicated patients, many of these rehabilitation goals have been managed before discharge.

For inpatients with severe complications and sequelae, additional temporary stays in skilled nursing facilities were especially helpful in the provision of a full range of services. Moreover, service to some of these outpatients is also affected. The patient might have a higher chance of being discharged without an optimal disposition having been generated, even if the rehabilitation team has been effective and efficient.

Within each rehabilitation team, one key solution is the mutual respect and regard for each member of the team. Mutual respect and professional behavior tend to combat the idea that one or another team member has shouldered most of the therapeutic burden for an inpatient. The team facilitator can also lead by example and regard. Consideration and tolerance are difficult to measure but important to rehabilitation team function. Goodwill and benevolence are nearly always relevant and useful for team collaboration.

DEALING WITH THE ARTIFICIAL FLOOR AND GLASS CEILING

The artificial floor robs the patient of necessary basic rehabilitation medicine services. Before progress toward acute rehabilitation goals can really take off, certain preliminary, basic management considerations that contribute in a significant way toward strengthening the patient should be implemented. These issues include safe eating, grooming, bed mobility, and needs communication. These issues are all usually managed through the composition of the rehabilitation team. Complications, such as falls, decubitus ulcers, urinary tract infections, or contractures, can be thoroughly evaluated and care initiated at a relatively early stage. Each of these areas is relatively underrepresented in current NS functional outcome scales. The measured rate of progress can, consequently, demonstrate a rather flat profile even when the patient is making good progress—the artificial floor. Problems arise when third-party payer gatekeepers demand discharge of these inpatients to extra care facilities (nursing homes) even though, with new funding methods, skilled nursing programs are limited in the care that they can provide.

The glass ceiling robs the patient and the family of effective follow-up monitoring and care. After acute rehabilitative progress has been made, some considerations are more difficult to solve than others. Included are usually housekeeping, equipment, and vocational issues. Each area is filled with details, forms, and the need for follow-up even under optimal circumstances. These areas are also usually underrepresented in NS functional outcome scales. Measured momentum demonstrates a digital plateau even though success in these three areas helps community re-entry programs—the glass ceiling. Third-party payer pressure has been to terminate the inpatient stay before these areas are satisfactorily managed. In theory, follow-up care could be provided on an outpatient basis, but in that case, the concentrated therapy needed is absent. If a patient is discharged with major problems in pain and weakness, the chances diminish that the patient will be able to master these three areas completely as an outpatient. Narrative documentation of team efforts is vital. Tips for careful narrative documentation include

1. Common goals and objectives should be present on each therapy or nursing note as well as in the narrative summary of the rehabilitation team meeting.

2. Impulsive, unclear, inconsistent narrative documentation can endanger an entire team's work.

3. Rehabilitation team members should communicate their findings and views on a daily basis.

4. Progress notes should reflect the common, active rehabilitation effort. Therapy notes in conflict with rehabilitation team goals are destructive and are usually recognized at some point.

5. Disputes arise, even in optimal circumstances. There is no regulation that every member of the rehabilitation team must be pleasant, even most of the time.

In fact, given the pervasive loss of privacy and the irritation and aggravation of constant, daily clinical or therapeutic demands, uncommon kindness, goodwill, and consideration are generously contributed within the rehabilitation team. Rehabilitation used to be placed in either an isolated location or in the basement. Modern facilities, though less depressing and better located to the mainstream of medical care, still help undermine an individual's privacy. Rehabilitation teams currently are responding positively even under disadvantageous conditions. Frequently, performance is above and beyond the call of duty.

We all should do our part. We all should communicate our needs within the team. We all should help other team members even before that help is formally requested. We all have to maintain a beneficial, good humored, and optimistic attitude. The whole rehabilitative effort can be twisted or wasted with a misdirected, negative attitude. Compromise and negotiation are far more efficient than confrontation between team members or between the team members and the patient or family.

EFFECT ON REHABILITATION

Many teams work together but often do not document that concerted action. Computer-friendly administrative forms have increased this problem in that narrative documentation has been replaced by forms emphasizing check-off boxes or fill-in-the-blank methodology. The dialogue within the rehabilitation medicine team, however, is not necessarily advanced by this methodology. In certain types of communication environments (e.g., some forms of computer electronic charts), it is less convenient and comfortable to access the comment section than the check-off box sections. An extra series of maneuvers must then be successfully negotiated for the person keying in the team conference note to get to the comment section. At certain rehabilitation centers, these notes are keyed in by computer analysts with little or no knowledge of the rehabilitation team process.

Realistically, narrative team progress notes still remain central to the justification to third-party payers of an individual patient's rehabilitation effort. Mathematical rating formulas, catch-up phone calls, letters, and e-mails do not adequately substitute. In addition, narrative notes should document the amount of neurologic return, the functional return, the goals, and the patient's response to therapy. These last areas are central to the whole rehabilitative program. Mathematical rating formulae at best seek to become the language for the rehabilitative team process, and many have undergone only superficial verification of such weak points as interval measurement. The narrative note should present the rehabilitation team's concerted efforts to manage rehabilitative challenges presented to the team. At the start of this chapter, some notice was given to these stroke patients' pain and weakness. Pain and weakness are managed within certain specific environments—the patient should be stroked and not stuck. Progress by the rehabilitation medicine team managing those challenges will not be effectively communicated without narrative progress notes.

Who will be keying in the rehabilitation medicine team progress notes? This function is a prerogative of the physician member of the team. It cannot be delegated, even to an attending resident physician. The physician member of the team should know what to do about rehabilitation challenges to the team. These physician members should familiarize themselves with what problems are being made manifest to the team before, during, and after team conferences so that troubleshooting can occur while the problems are smaller and easier to manage—not after they become large and complex obstructions. It is the team physician leader's thoughts, ideas, and plans that third-party carriers want communicated. Physician members can present role models to resident physicians, but the fundamental responsibility to facilitate team functions cannot and must not be delegated. Rehabilitation medicine teams should continually be built and maintained. These are also functions of the physician team member. These functions can be shared with other team members so that optimal effective participation of every team member is assured.

It is possible to have too many team conferences. These conferences are expensive and add to overhead costs even under optimal conditions. Too many meetings take everyone away from therapy for long periods. A symptom of this situation is when many, if not most, of the presentations at the team conference are made by substitutes—not by the clinician actually treating the patient. The difficulty that arises is that these substitutes cannot answer questions but must pass along comments to the treating clinician for the rest of the team. One important goal of rehabilitation teams, and the solution to this specific difficulty, is to make every minute count. In that way, only the regularly scheduled fortnightly or weekly conferences are really necessary. Attendance at these conferences would then probably improve. Extra admission or discharge conferences would be less relevant and less necessary, as they would be accommodated within regular team conferences and team communication outside of team meetings.

REFERENCES

1. Campbell JN. Nerve lesions and the generation of pain. *Muscle Nerve* 2001;24:1261–1273.
2. Campbell JN, Long DM. Peripheral nerve stimulation in the treatment of intractable pain. *J Neurosurg* 1976;45:692–699.
3. Campbell JN, *et al*. Myelinated afferents signal the hyperalgesia associated with nerve injury. *Pain* 1988;32:89–94.
4. Koltzenberg M, *et al*. Dynamic and static components of mechanical hyperalgesia in human hairy skin. *Pain* 1992;51:207–219.
5. Ochoa JL, Yarnitsky D. Mechanical hyperalgesias in neuropathic pain patients. *Ann Neurol* 1993;33:465–472.
6. Price DD, *et al*. Sensory testing of pathophysiological mechanisms of pain in patients with reflex sympathetic dystrophy. *Pain* 1992;49:163–173.
7. Treede R-D, Cole JD. Dissociated secondary hyperalgesia in a subject with large fiber sensory neuropathy. *Pain* 1993;53:169–174.
8. Cervero F, *et al*. A psychophysical study of secondary hyperalgesia. *Pain* 1994; 58:21–28.
9. LaMotte RH, Campbell JN. Comparison of responses of warm and nociceptive C-fiber afferents in monkey with human judgements of thermal pain. *J Neurophysiol* 1978;41:509–528.
10. LaMotte RH, *et al*. Neurogenic hyperalgesia. *J Neurophysiol* 1991;66:190–211.
11. Baker NB, Baker LH. *Clinical Neurology*. Philadelphia: J.B. Lippincott, 1988.
12. Batterham RW, *et al*. Can we achieve accountability for long term outcomes? *Arch Phys Med Rehabil* 1996;77:1219–1225.
13. Benson DF, Ardila A. *Aphasia*. New York: Oxford University Press, 1996.
14. Bougouslavsky J, Regli F. Anterior cerebral artery territory infarction in the Lausanne Stroke Registry. *Arch Neurol* 1990;47:144–148.
15. Cook L, Smith DS, Truman G. Using functional independence profiles as an index of outcome in the rehabilitation of brain injured patients. *Arch Phys Med Rehabil* 1994;75:390–393.
16. Gacs G, *et al*. Occurrence and mechanism of occlusion of the anterior cerebral artery. *Stroke* 1983;14:952–959.
17. Gelmers HJ. Non-paralytic motor disturbances and speech disorders. *J Neurol Neurosurg Psychiatry* 1983;46:1052–1059.

18. Grimby G, *et al*. Structure of a combination of functional independence measure and instrumental activity measure items in community-living persons. *Arch Phys Med Rehabil* 1996;77:1109–1114.
19. Harvey RF, *et al*. Patient profiles. *Arch Phys Med Rehabil* 1983;64:268–271.
20. Kazui S, *et al*. A clinical study of patients with cerebral infarction localized in the territory of the anterior cerebral artery. *Jpn J Stroke* 1987;9:317–319.
21. Ottenbacher KJ, *et al*. The reliability of functional independence measure. *Arch Phys Med Rehabil* 1996;77:1226–1232.
22. Pruitt SD, *et al*. Functional status in children with limb deficiency. *Arch Phys Med Rehabil* 1996;77:1233–1238.
23. Stineman MG, *et al*. Four methods for characterizing disability in the formation of function related groups. *Arch Phys Med Rehabil* 1994;75:1277–1283.
24. Stineman MG, *et al*. The functional independence measure. *Arch Phys Med Rehabil* 1996;77:1101–1108.
25. The Center for Functional Assessment Research and the Uniform Data System for Medical Rehabilitation. GUIDE for use of the Uniform Data Set for Medical Rehabilitation including the Functional Independence Measure (FIM), Version 3.0. Buffalo, N.Y: Research Foundation, State University of New York at Buffalo, 1990.

8 Adjustment to Disability

Candia P. Kaplan

Studies indicate quality-of-life and functional outcomes reported by stroke survivors were comparable regardless of whether the stroke was due to infarction or hemorrhage.[1,2] However, survivors of hemorrhagic strokes appear to make gains at a faster rate.[3] Throughout recovery, stroke survivors and their families typically undergo a process of adjustment to disability that can be facilitated by a rehabilitation psychologist.

Admission to a rehabilitation hospital may precipitate distress, particularly in older persons who may have difficulty adjusting to the expectations for active participation and the ethic that guides the rehabilitative process. The rehabilitation ethic supports independent function, active participation on the part of the patient and his or her family, cooperation, acceptance of pain, and progress toward clinical goals.[4] When patients do not appear to conform to this ethic, psychologists can identify the barriers to full participation, explore values, and facilitate the rehabilitative process via education, counseling, and/or behavioral management. Adults who enter a rehabilitation setting may have been socialized to a more passive role as to what is expected from a "good patient" and may benefit from an awareness of the unique demands of rehabilitation. Younger patients tend to be more upset about physical change, such as facial droop, and they may refuse to look at themselves in the mirror. Acceptance from peers usually is helpful. Existential psychotherapy focused on personal identity, the process of becoming, and the meaning of life may be particularly beneficial. Those persons with a strong religious background may think that their life was spared for a reason and may therefore be open to new possibilities and goals.

Conventional wisdom might indicate that new symptoms, such as insomnia and decreased appetite, would be symptoms of clinical depression. However, it is important to realize that symptoms might not have the same diagnostic accuracy in a stroke survivor.[5] Post-stroke hypoarousal (i.e., slowed motor speed, slowed mental processing, slumped posture, or frequent yawning) may manifest as symptoms that would be indicative of depression in a psychiatrically ill person.[6] In addition, misattributions about the cause of stroke can negatively affect the emotions within the family and are often amenable to intervention. Guilt for not getting the stroke survivor to an emergency room soon enough for the administration of tissue plasminogen activator is a new cause of depressive symptoms and can be reduced via education and cognitive behavioral therapy.

The loss of independence and need to rely on others for basic life functions, such as eating, bathing, dressing, and, especially, elimination, creates a sometimes frightening and demoralizing situation for patients. Personal care from an individual who is not the patient's sex can elicit negative reactions based on modesty or can elicit re-experiencing feelings of helplessness and fear in persons who may have been abused in the past. They may benefit from interventions provided by a psychologist who is of the same sex. Often, older adults report feeling worthless if they are dependent in activities of daily life and cannot be as productive as they were before their stroke. Supportive therapy can help tease apart personal worth from productivity and independence. Often, an exploration of productivity from a life span approach is helpful. Similarly, if a patient can report being lovable and worthy as an infant or young child when they were not engaged in productive work, then it may be easier to accept worthiness as inherent in the individual rather than just the product of work. Adjusting to disability and loss of function while simultaneously adjusting to the patient role can be a difficult process. The rehabilitation psychologist is uniquely qualified to address these concerns.

Language and visual impairments can contribute to anxiety and depression. It is difficult to measure depressive symptoms in persons with aphasia. Those with expressive aphasia may exaggerate nonverbal gestures to convey information. However, they may be able to point to a visual analog scale or make a choice between a happy and sad face. If they are able to reliably respond to a yes/no format, the Mood Assessment Scale may be used.[7] Clinical lore used to be that persons with left hemispheric strokes were more likely to experience depressive spectrum disorders than those with right hemispheric strokes. However, lateralization effects for the prevalence of depression in stroke survivors are not always found.[8] The unanticipated precipitous decline in control over bodily functions, cognitive impairments that make thinking an exhausting process, new visual limitations in an unfamiliar environment, and struggles with communication deficits are frightening experiences. Anxious feelings may precede or co-exist with depressive reactions. A calm, patient-centered therapeutic relationship can reduce levels of anxiety. Group therapy can help develop an awareness of clinical improvements, as patients who are further along in their recovery often can recognize improvements in other patients on the rehabilitation unit. Non-professional stroke survivors who function as co-therapists can help model a positive attitude via functionally independent role models.

Adaptation to an altered physical appearance may depend on prior emotional status, level of self-esteem, and whether the patient feels unconditional acceptance in significant relationships. Older age, committed relationships, and financial stability may be protective factors. The presence of strong spiritual beliefs may either protect against depressive reactions or contribute to guilty feelings. Occasionally, the rehabilitation psychologist encounters patients who have experienced clinical depression because they believe that if they were truly committed to their faith, they would not have experienced a stroke. It is as if their physical symptoms are an outward manifestation of impiety or immorality for which they are being punished. Since publication of Freud's *Mourning and Melancholia*,[9] disturbed self-regard has been a recognized clinical symptom that has distinguished grief from depression. Recent empirical findings support a theoretical differentiation of grief and depression, with guilt a differentiating factor.[10,11] When patients complain of religiously based guilt, cognitive-behavioral and/or existential therapy and collaboration with a chaplain are indicated.

Similarly, the interdisciplinary team members may have concerns regarding the patient's mood. Frequently, psychologists are consulted after therapist observations of patient tears; overheard comments regarding futility, loss, or sadness; poor appetite; refusal of therapies; and apathy. Not all of these symptoms are indicative of clinical depression. A psychological consultation elucidates the unique pre-morbid characteristics of the patient and the support system, injury characteristics, and presenting symptoms. Usually, sudden tears that disappear after distraction are more indicative of lability from organic brain injury. Patients benefit from normalization of the crying episodes as well as from interventions that offer distraction techniques to control crying. It is helpful to ask the patient to look at something nearby and ask questions about the object as a distraction. The patient may be surprised to see their tears go away within the first minute that they participate in such an activity. The family usually is relieved to learn that the patient has organic lability that can be expected to have reduced frequency and duration. Sometimes, sadness in stroke survivors is indicative of a grief reaction focused on the recent losses sustained as a consequence of a stroke. They miss the person they once were. In this case, intervention is focused on facilitating the grief process.[12] A developmental approach can also help integrate transitions across the life span. Reactive depressive symptoms are not just the consequences of the stroke itself. Rejection or abandonment by significant others, loss of the ability to carry on life roles in the family and community, financial worries, and sexual concerns can contribute to a depressive reaction. If the patient's symptoms meet diagnostic criteria for a depressive disorder, appropriate psychological interventions and medication are indicated. Depending on factors such as current symptoms and prior psychiatric history, an evaluation for appropriate medication includes consideration of stimulants, antidepressants, and anticonvulsants.

Goal setting is expected in a rehabilitation setting. It is important that the psychologist encourage active patient participation in goal setting, because research has shown that hope can be operationalized as the ability to set meaningful goals along with the belief that the individual has the means to achieve his or her goals.[13,14] Increasing evidence suggests mediational factors, such as hope, are more critical than life events in predicting adjustment.

Energy level, sensory changes, impaired bladder and bowel function, and altered body image can diminish desire for sex after stroke. In addition, partners can fear that intercourse will cause another stroke. It is important to remember that sexual problems are multifactorial and include co-morbid medical and psychological conditions. Patients' sexual concerns may include worry that others will not find them attractive or desirable after the stroke.[15] Altered self-image can be addressed via reassurance regarding acceptance, performance, and safety. The focus can be shifted from physical attractiveness to more intrinsic and permanent aspects of the self. Greater sexual difficulty has been observed in persons with left hemispheric strokes than in right, indicating the impact of language and the importance of removing barriers to communication. Movement limitations due to motor impairments can require adjustments. Bodily changes also can result in fears that sexual function will be impossible. Specific concerns can be elicited in the context of a supportive professional relationship. Modifications of sexual behaviors can be suggested by the psychologist. Should the patient prefer a therapist of another sex, consultative arrangements or the assistance of a nurse can be arranged. The best predictor of resumption of sexual activity has been higher frequency of sexual activity before having a stroke.

In time, with adequate intervention, stroke survivors may come to view their condition as no more disruptive than any other bodily condition, even though residual physical sequelae remain and society may still treat them as if they are handicapped or aged. Patients who have sustained a stroke may express positive feelings about themselves when they have begun to feel they are a competent and adequate survivor rather than a victim.[16]

Because persons seen in rehabilitation facilities are a microcosm of the world at large, it is not unusual that family issues may surround and impede the process of rehabilitation and discharge back to the community. Marital stress may increase after the serious illness of one partner. Occasionally, the treatment team may have concerns about the partner's ability or interest in caring for the patient. Alternately, the identified family member may find his or her schedule is too busy to enable him or her to show up for family training necessary for the patient to be discharged. For relatively minor problems, brief marital therapy and information may be all that is needed to engage the partner in the rehabilitation process or to facilitate discharge plans. Affordable home modification or assistance also may relieve partner concerns and increase a sense of self-efficacy in the ability to care for the patient on discharge.

Unhealthy pre-morbid lifestyles, including poor diet, smoking, and inadequate exercise, may be addressed while the patient is in acute rehabilitation. Often, the reality of physical impairment is sufficient to motivate patient cooperation with lifestyle modifications. Follow-up for the outpatient phase of recovery may be arranged through the continuum of care before discharge from acute rehabilitation.

Because acute medical rehabilitation hospital stays are significantly shorter, persons with stroke probably have not had the opportunity to learn how their stroke may have affected their daily life. Often, it is not until discharge that they find limitations imposed by stroke sequelae. Persons who have experienced a stroke are frequently affected by slowed speed of mental processing and response. Many patients find they must laboriously think through processes that once were automatic. They feel unsure of themselves and their abilities. This can contribute to frustration as well as a shaken sense of themselves. Continued frustration, social isolation, changed roles, and unemployment can result in depressive disorders after discharge from acute rehabilitation. It is crucial that continued rehabilitation psychology services remain available after discharge.

Depressive symptoms after discharge are more likely to be functional than organic as new limitations and barriers to full participation in the community are encountered outside the hospital. In the worst-case scenario, persons who are unable to accept bodily changes after stroke may attempt suicide. Depression is treatable, with resultant improvement in the quality of life. Older individuals have responded well to cognitive-behavioral therapy, which has the advantage of reduced treatment side effects. Additionally, behavioral interventions can reduce stress and hypertension that are believed to contribute to hemorrhagic stroke. This is important to reduce the likelihood of rebleed and consequent additional impairments. Psychological assessment and treatment as needed through the lifetime also can reduce excessive medical costs by promoting healthier lifestyles and improved medical compliance.[17]

For some individuals who are recovering from stroke, return to meaningful activity is a significant concern. It is important to protect their insurance resources and withhold formal neuropsychological assessment until sufficient recovery has occurred to determine whether return to work or school is a realistic treatment goal. In the meantime, increased leisure activities can provide important socialization, reduce the likelihood of depression, and ensure respite for care providers. The frequency and complexity of activities should be commensurate with the patient's level of energy. Additional rest periods may facilitate greater participation. Likewise, the amount of environmental stimulation should be monitored. Patients may be more sensitive to, and distracted by, noise and visual clutter after stroke. Likewise, they may be less able to process new verbal or visual-spatial information, depending on the site of brain injury. Relative strengths in one processing modality can be used to facilitate cognitive processing in the other modality. Some patients are able to discover useful strengths for themselves; however, maximal return of function can be attained with the appropriate professional interventions provided by occupational, speech, and psychological therapists.

Return to the community provides another key time when patients realize change in their social roles. For persons who valued work or the money they were able to provide to their family, or both, time off from work or early retirement and inability to function in the same manner can be serious blows to their sense of well-being. Some question the reason for their survival and may require assistance to identify the unique answer to their quest for a meaningful role in their family and a purpose in living. This is particularly so if they are worried about how the family can deal with the cost of their treatment.

Rehabilitation psychologists hold a unique position on the interdisciplinary team throughout the continuity of care. They respond to a wider range of needs and barriers to return function than just patients' physical status or functional independence. Rehabilitation psychologists address problems in mood, attitude, behavior, and personal and family adjustment as they relate to participation in the rehabilitation setting or discharge plans. The scope of interventions includes, but is not limited to, psychological assessment, counseling or psychotherapy, pain management, family education, behavioral management, and vocational counseling. Rehabilitation psychologists also address barriers to meaningful integration back into the community. Rehabilitation psychologists are specifically trained to evaluate and treat the short- and long-term psychosocial consequences of hemorrhagic stroke.[18]

They use a holistic perspective that emphasizes optimal use of a patient's strengths to address limitations arising from disability. In addition to direct delivery of psychological services, they conduct research that helps determine recovery parameters to better counsel patients and their families about expectations for recovery or remediation of cognitive deficits, or both.[19] Research can also guide interventions to better address emotional consequences of stroke on patients and care providers. Psychologists have used expertise in research methodology, physiology, and behavior to develop and evaluate new treatments such as constraint-induced movement.[20]

Rehabilitation psychologists function in both inpatient and outpatient settings. In the acute hospital setting, rehabilitation psychologists often screen for mental status and behavior as they relate to rehabilitation potential. Early psycho-educational counseling for the patient and family is important in setting appropriate expectations and facilitating adjustment to disability.

REFERENCES

1. Bamford J, et al. A 3-year longitudinal study. Stroke 1996;27:270–275.
2. de Hann RJ, et al. Quality of life after stroke. Impact of stroke type and lesion location. Stroke 1995;26:402–408.
3. Chae J, et al. Functional outcome of hemorrhagic and nonhemorrhagic stroke patients after in-patient rehabilitation. Am J Phys Med Rehabil 1996;75:177–182.
4. Wegener ST. The rehabilitation ethic and ethics. Rehabil Psychol 1996;41:3–17.
5. Woessner R, Caplan B. Emotional distress following stroke: Interpretive limitations of the SCL–90-R. Assessment 1996;3:291–305.
6. Ross ED, Rush J. Diagnosis and neuroanatomical correlates of depression in brain-damaged patients. Arch Gen Psychiatry 1981;38:1344–1354.
7. Yesavage JA, et al. Development and validation of a geriatric depression screening scale: A preliminary report. J Psychiatr Res 1983;17:37–49.
8. Gordon W, et al. Issues in the diagnosis of post-stroke depression. Rehabil Psychol 1991;35:71–87.
9. Freud S. Mourning and Melancholia. In: J Strachey (ed and trans.), The Standard Edition of the Complete Works of Sigmund Freud, Vol. 14. London: Hogarth Press, 1957.
10. Breckenridge JN, et al. Characteristic depressive symptoms of bereaved elders. J Gerontol 1986;41:163–168.
11. Kaplan CP, Gallagher-Thompson D. Treatment of clinical depression in caregivers of spouses with dementia. J Cogn Psychother 1995;9:35–44.
12. Worden JW. Grief Counseling and Grief Therapy: A Handbook for the Mental Health Practitioner, second edition. New York: Springer, 1991.
13. Snyder CR. The Psychology of Hope. New York: Free Press, 1994.
14. McDermott D, Snyder CR. Making Hope Happen. Oakland, CA: New Harbinger Publications, 1999.
15. Trilok NM. Sexuality post stroke. Phys Med Rehabil 1993;7:225–236.

16. Payne EC, *et al.* Goal directedness and older-adult adjustment. *J Counsel Psychol* 1991;38:302–308.
17. Cummings N. *Biodyne Training Manual of Brief, Intermittent Psychotherapy Throughout the Life Cycle.* San Francisco: Biodyne Institute, 1983.
18. Patterson DR, Hanson SL. Joint Division 22 and ACRM Guidelines for post-doctoral training in Rehabilitation Psychology. *Rehabil Psychol* 1995;40: 299–310.
19. DeLuca J, Diamond BJ. Aneurysm of the anterior communicating artery: A review of neuroanatomical and neuropsychological sequelae. *J Clin Exp Neuropsychol* 1995;17:100–121.
20. Taub E, *et al.* Constraint-induced movement therapy: A new approach to treatment in physical medicine and rehabilitation. *Rehabil Psychol* 1998;43:152–170.

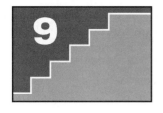

Complications: Rebleeding, Hydrocephalus, and Delayed Cerebral Ischemia

Paul E. Kaplan

With enhanced radiologic and technological methodology, more and more scanning equipment is being directed at the cause and evolution of stroke syndromes. For example, a recent study applied computed tomography (CT) or magnetic resonance imaging (MRI), carotid duplex ultrasonography, and transesophageal echocardiography to determining the prognosis of lacunar strokes.[1] Additionally, MRI methodology has also been used to generate stroke evolution models,[2] and diffusion-perfusion MRIs have delineated perihematomal hypoperfusion around intracranial hemorrhages with poor outcomes.[3] MRIs have delineated silent strokes[4] and criteria associated with depression after strokes.[5] Using this methodology, it was possible to demonstrate that deep cerebral infarcts extend as far as subinsular regions[6] and to associate movement disorders with specific thalamic strokes.[7]

MRI has not been the only scanning method used to investigate stroke disorders. Positron emission tomography scans have been used to document the coexistence of Alzheimer's disease and strokes in patients with early progressive dementia,[8] and the coexistence of stroke and vascular dementia.[9] However, the full potential of this line of study can be glimpsed in an investigation of stroke patients undergoing arm training.[10] An impression can be formed of the type of brain reorganization required for this rehabilitative activity. All of the complications noted in this chapter are diagnosed earlier and more accurately than ever before through the use of scanning techniques.[11-25]

REBLEEDING

The true incidence of rebleeding—particularly of seepage rather than frank hemorrhage—will probably never be known. Reported rebleeding varies from 20% to 40% and commonly occurs within 24 hours of ictus.[11,16,19] Additionally, the risk of this complication remains high for 2 more weeks. During this period, physical and emotional stress factors (see Chapter 1) should be reduced as much as possible. Even afterward, the threat of rebleeding, though reduced, is still a prominent complication. Rebleeding can promote the formation of added glial tissue, late seizure disorders, frontal lobe syndrome onset, personality change, and cognitive decline.

On the other hand, too much inactivity only augments deconditioning. Muscular atrophy, joint contractures, decubitus ulcers, deep vein thrombophlebitis, and kidney stones often accompany deconditioning. This special situation often makes rehabilitation during these 2 weeks difficult, and special therapeutic prescription writing and team planning are necessary. Certainly, monitoring pulse and blood pressure during therapy would be advantageous. Antifibrinolytics reduce rebleeding but also increase the risk of two other major complications—hydrocephalus and delayed cerebral ischemia.

HYDROCEPHALUS

Etiology

Hydrocephalus is a specific cause of organic brain syndrome and associated dementia that can be treated. When treated in an effective and timely manner, dementia is partially or completely reversible. Hydrocephalus is an occasional complication of hemorrhagic stroke disorders. Under favorable circumstances, hydrocephalus is one of the few causes of dementia that is reversible. If the hydrocephalus is of short duration, does not increase intracerebral ventricular fluid pressure, and is not associated with marked or severe dementia, reversing the hydrocephalus might also reverse these patients' dementia. Therefore, diagnosis and treatment of hydrocephalus becomes more important than statistics alone would indicate to the management of patients with hemorrhagic stroke.

Hydrocephalus is not caused by one specific factor. It is the common result of a heterogeneous group of injuries and disorders. Any inflammation, insult, infection, ischemia, infarction, or surgical procedure involving the central nervous system can subsequently generate inflammation of the tissue surrounding the few small outlets from the ventricles to the subarachnoid space so that those outlets are effectively rendered dysfunctional (Figure 9.1).

Before CT and MRI scans, diagnosis was made by pneumoencephalography. If air passed from the ventricles to the subarachnoid

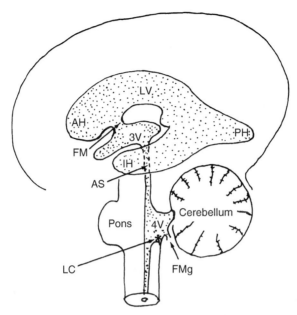

Figure 9.1 The ventricular network of the cerebral hemispheres is depicted. Note that these ventricles have only two relatively small outlets to the spinal portions of the cerebrospinal fluid system. These two outlets are situated quite near vascular tissues and are both strategic and vulnerable to inflammation. (AH = anterior horn; AS = cerebral aqueduct; FM = foramen of Monro; FMg = foramen of Magendie; IH = inferior horn; LC = foramen of Luschka; LV = lateral ventricle; PH = posterior horn; 3V = third ventricle; 4V = fourth ventricle.) (Reprinted with permission from Cailliet R. *Pain: Mechanisms and Management*. Philadelphia: F.A. Davis, 1993;35.)

space, the hydrocephalus was stated to be nonobstructive or communicating. If air did not pass, the hydrocephalus was said to be obstructive or noncommunicating.[12,21] At this point, as new fluid collects in the ventricular system in the limited space of the cranial vault, the cerebral hemispheres are placed in a condition of physical and vascular stress by an expanding mass. The gray and white matter of those cerebral hemispheres become ischemic as that matter is physically pressed by the fluid collection.

Onset and Presentation

Hydrocephalus is not like ictus nor traumatic brain injury in which cases one can pinpoint a particular date and time of onset. Its onset is gradual, insidious, and partial in nature. That makes hydrocephalus harder to detect at an early stage. In adults after hemorrhagic stroke, headaches, neck and back pain, and ophthalmologic signs and symptoms are the earliest evidences. None of these are specific for hydrocephalus.

Even with normal-pressure hydrocephalus, as the amount of fluid grows, deficits can increase from intermittent failures of concentration, increased irritability, intermittent obtundation, memory deficits, and coma. Simultaneously, the onset of hypertension and frontal lobe syndrome have been observed. At a severe and advanced state, gait disorders, urinary incontinence, and a fully expressed organic brain syndrome are usually noted.[5,8,10,13] Hydrocephalus with increased intracerebral intraventricular pressure produces a more accelerated, irreversible, severe accumulation of the deficits previously noted. These patterns can mimic certain aspects of those deficits observed with brain tumors or any space-occupying intracerebral lesion.

Apraxic and aphasic disorders can also be present but are evidently not frequent throughout much of the clinical spectrum. The key clinical pattern most commonly noted is deficits of attention and cognition more severe and out of all proportion to any mild, focal sensory or motor deficits. Complications of pneumoencephalography can be severe, but CT and MRI scan technology has made the diagnosis of hydrocephalus much easier. With routine postoperative therapeutic protocols, this complication is now routinely detected.

As these signs and symptoms progress, the patient often reaches a therapeutic plateau despite intensive therapy or may even regress. Instruction given even daily will not be carried over to the next therapeutic session. After medical or surgical therapy of the hydrocephalus, however, the patient can make even faster progress than noted before the condition arose. However, this condition can return. With each new treatment, the progress made is usually reduced. But for those with only one episode of hydrocephalus, detected early and aggressively treated, dementia can resolve and not return. When this special result is seen, it can be gratifying. This clinical situation is probably unique to this complication.

DELAYED CEREBRAL ISCHEMIA

Onset

Delayed cerebral ischemia is usually a serious, intensive complication that is destructive to that patient's rehabilitation potential. So far, the focus of this chapter has been on hemorrhagic stroke. In delayed cerebral ischemia, usually 10 days after the neurosurgical procedure has been performed, the patient experiences the rapid, sudden onset of a severe, new ictal episode of thrombotic stroke.[22]

This complication is rare in the presence of an unruptured intracranial aneurysm. It is usually preceded by vasospasm that is usually related to the quantity of subarachnoid blood seen on the CT scan.[23-25] A number of factors have been associated with it.[11-17] These factors include, but are not limited to, hydrocephalus, hypotension during surgery, and hyponatremia. Dense hemiplegia, hemianesthesia, central facial palsy, cognitive deficits, apraxia, and aphasia are often noted. Unlike hemorrhagic stroke, once observed, these signs and symptoms frequently do not spontaneously resolve.[17-19]

Treatment

Treatment options have included, but have not been limited to, blood pressure elevation, hypervolemia, endovascular balloon angioplasty, and intra-arterial papaverine infusions.[13-15,22-25] Although some of the physical deficits can be modified with the vigorous medical treatment noted above, cognitive deficits are commonly resistant to this medical treatment.[13-15,17-25]

Once this complication has occurred, a combination of therapy, psychotherapy, and psychotropic medication is indicated; however, prevention is optimal. Moreover, once this complication has become evident, the likelihood of the patient developing dementia is augmented, and the possibilities of achieving safe, independent functional activities usually decline. As the patient's rehabilitation potential becomes progressively limited, discharge to some form of assisted living environment becomes more probable. However, the existence of more effective monitoring devices and vasolytic treatment choices might augment the possibility of effective prevention in the future.

EFFECT ON REHABILITATION

The specific complications noted in this chapter can be separate or combined. Hemorrhagic strokes in patients with cerebral aneurysms can be associated with conditions of delayed cerebral ischemia. One complication can help generate the others. Rebleeding can contribute to the risk of these patients developing hydrocephalus. The great end result of either type of combination is progressive dementia—dementia that, depending on the cause, could be treated. The consequences of these complications are great, as the patient's functional ability is often severely limited. Activities of daily living, transfer activities in bed or out of bed, and social rapport and communication are all vulnerable to cognitive decline. For the neuropsychological aspects of these patients, please see Chapter 10. It is more difficult to care for a demented patient.

Without careful, tender, patient care, the patient's life expectancy is reduced.

Other assorted complications, such as falls, burns, and decubitus ulcers, are common. These miscellaneous complications lead to contractures, fractures, and pulmonary emboli. They do not lead to the difficult rehabilitation obstacle of dementia. Instead of cognitive deterioration, increased physical functional burdens of mobility, hygiene, and self-sufficiency are present. These heterogeneous complications do generally respond to either prevention or early treatment. However, a high index of differential diagnostic sensitivity is necessary so that these complications can be prevented before they occur. When physical complications have been allowed to persist for some time, they have a tendency to generate permanent impairment and increase patient disability, with diminished quality of life. Because inactivity is also associated with morbidity and mortality, these physical complications also eventually shorten the length of the patient's life.

REFERENCES

1. Kasui S, *et al.* Lacunar stroke. *Cerebrovasc Dis* 2001;12:325–330.
2. Rose SE, *et al.* MRI based diffusion and perfusion predictive model to estimate stroke evolution. *Magn Reson Imaging* 2001;19:1043–1053.
3. Kidwell CS, *et al.* Diffusion-perfusion MR evaluation of perihematomal injury in hyperacute intracerebral hemorrhage. *Neurology* 2001;57:1611–1617.
4. Bernick C, *et al.* Silent MRI infarcts and the risk of future stroke. *Neurology* 2001;57:1222–1229.
5. Vataja R, *et al.* Magnetic resonance imaging correlates of depression after ischemic stroke. *Arch Gen Psychiatry* 2001;58:925–931.
6. Wong EH, *et al.* Deep cerebral infarcts extending to the subinsular region. *Stroke* 2001;32:2272–2277.
7. Lehericy S, *et al.* Clinical characteristics and topography of lesions in movement disorders due to thalamic lesions. *Neurology* 2001;57:1055–1066.
8. Silverman DH, *et al.* Positron emission tomography in evaluation of dementia. *JAMA* 2001;286:2120–2127.
9. De Reuck J, *et al.* Cobalt-55 positron emission tomography in vascular dementia. *J Neurol Sci* 2001;193:1–6.
10. Nelles G, *et al.* Arm training induced brain plasticity in stroke studied with serial positron emission tomography. *Neuroimage* 2001;13:1146–1154.
11. Ausman JI, *et al.* Current management of cerebral aneurysms. *Surg Neurol* 1985;24:625–635.
12. Benzel EC, *et al.* Communicating hydrocephalus in adults. *Neurosurgery* 1990;26:655–660.
13. Buchheit F, Boyer P. Review of treatment of symptomatic cerebral vasospasm with nimodipine. *Acta Neurochir* 1988;Suppl45:51–55.
14. Gilsbach JM. Nimodipine in the prevention of ischaemic deficits after aneurysmal subarachnoid hemorrhage. *Acta Neurochir* 1988;Suppl45:41–50.

15. Hijdra A, *et al.* Aneurysmal subarachnoid hemorrhage. *Stroke* 1987;18: 1061–1067.
16. Kassell NJ, Torner JC. Aneurysmal rebleeding. *Neurosurgery* 1983;13:179–181.
17. Mendelow AD. Pathophysiology of delayed ischaemic dysfunction after subarachnoid hemorrhage. *Acta Neurochir* 1988;Suppl45:7–10.
18. Mysiw WJ, Jackson RD. Relationship of new onset systemic hypertension and normal pressure hydrocephalus. *Brain Injury* 1990;4:233–238.
19. Popovic EA, Siu K. Ruptured intracranial aneurysms. *Med J Aust* 1989;150:492–501.
20. Ropper AH, Zervas NT. Outcome one year after SAH from cerebral aneurysm. *J Neurosurg* 1984;60:909–915.
21. Russell D. *Observations on the Pathology of Hydrocephalus.* London: Medical Research Council Special Report Series No 265, Her Majesty's Stationary Office, 1949.
22. Schievink W1. Intracranial aneurysms. *N Engl J Med* 1997;336:28–40.
23. Story PB. Psychiatric sequelae of subarachnoid hemorrhage. *BMJ* 1967;3:261–266.
24. Sundt TM, *et al.* Results and complications of surgical management of 809 intracranial aneurysms in 722 cases. *J Neurosurg* 1982;56:753–755.
25. Weir B, MacDonald L. Cerebral vasospasm. *Clin Neurosurg* 1993;40:40–55.

10 Neuropsychological Factors in Stroke

Candia P. Kaplan

Neuropsychologists focus on brain–behavior relationships. Consequently, they evaluate behavioral correlates of hemorrhagic stroke by observation and objective assessment. Serial assessment can monitor cognitive status and demonstrate improvement or deterioration. The specific deficits experienced by survivors of hemorrhagic stroke depend on the location, severity, and number of focal lesions. Taken as a diverse group, survivors of hemorrhagic stroke have better outcomes than those with ischemic stroke. If there is no intrinsic brain injury, blood resorbs over time, and patients can experience a rather rapid recovery. If there are residual disabilities, the pattern of impairment varies with the etiology and location of the hemorrhage.

Although the pathogenic course and symptoms differ for ischemic and hemorrhagic stroke, the traditional separation between these two types of stroke may be an oversimplification. Some obstructions to blood flow are hemorrhagic in nature, whereas some hemorrhagic strokes result in vasospasm, which impedes blood flow and can create focal infarction. Therefore, hemorrhagic stroke can be broadly used as a model for all strokes.

Intracerebral hemorrhage (ICH) most commonly is the consequence of ruptured blood vessels at the base of the cortex, with brain injury usually in subcortical structures (i.e., basal ganglia, thalamus, and brain stem). Hypertension is a common cause of ICH. Survivors' abilities can range from functional independence to the permanent vegetative state. Chronic oral anticoagulants also can contribute to strokes if they are not well controlled. Others develop ICH due to weakened walls of small vessels from lipohyalinosis.[1] The second most frequent cause of ICH is arteriovenous malformation (congenitally abnormal tangle of vessels that can rupture). These patients tend to be younger. Elderly patients can present with ICH due to amyloid angiopathy, a degenerative disorder of blood vessels associated with Alzheimer's disease. Persons with impaired blood clotting from hemophilia, acquired liver disease, or medications such as aspirin and warfarin (Coumadin) represent a fourth group that can develop ICH. Most ICHs present with symptoms that differ from ischemic strokes. First, they do not usually occur in traditional vascular territories like the middle cerebral artery. Instead, ICH more commonly occurs in the basal ganglia and brain stem, with only 22% lobar and another 8% cerebellar.[2] When an ICH does occur in the middle cerebral artery territory, it may extend beyond the traditional boundary.

Clinical ICH symptoms may be more diverse and appear as a combination of signs of increased intracerebral pressure as well as symptoms produced by ischemic strokes in various vascular territories. Features reflect the location, size, direction of parenchymal extension, and ventricular involvement. In contrast with ICH, in which the mortality is low but morbidity high, many patients with subarachnoid hemorrhage (SAH) do not survive. The most common cause of SAH is an aneurysm, usually arising at branching sites of large arteries in the circle of Willis.[2] Bleeding is vigorous and under arterial pressure. Ruptured aneurysms usually occur in persons between 40 and 70 years old.[1] The second leading cause of SAH is arteriovenous malformations. Initial symptoms include severe headache, vomiting, somnambulance, and altered consciousness. Focal signs are usually absent initially but can arise from the pressure of blood in the cisterns pressing on cranial nerves or adjacent structures. Furthermore, complications of SAH include rebleeding, obstructive hydrocephalus, and seizures. Those most likely to experience SAH from ruptured vascular malformations are women in their 20s and 30s, most commonly during pregnancy and delivery.

The most difficult cognitive and behavioral recovery is often seen in persons who have sustained an aneurysmic rupture of the anterior communicating artery (ACoA). Neurobehavioral changes, collectively called the *ACoA syndrome*, include amnesia, confabulation, executive dysfunction, and personality change. A patient may manifest all of these deficits in varying degrees of severity together or in isolation.[1] The syndrome occurs in up to 56% of cases around the time of rehabilitation hospitalization; however, prevalence drops to approximately 15% in the years post surgery.[3] The ACoA syndrome is the likely result of vasospasm and infarction after aneurysm clipping. Because the ACoA, anterior cerebral artery, and recurrent artery of Heubner can be affected by postsurgical vasospasm, brain areas supplied by these vessels can undergo infarction secondary to vasospasm.[1] The ACoA supplies the basal forebrain, which includes the nucleus basalis of Meynert and septal nuclei, which are involved in memory. The anterior cerebral artery supplies the orbital and medial frontal areas, which are believed to mediate emotional behavior. The recurrent artery of Heubner supplies the caudate nuclei. Memory impairments include anterograde amnesia for new information and a temporally graded retrograde amnesia in which older memories are recalled better than more recent information. The executive dysfunction includes lack of awareness, poor initiation, apathy, impaired abstract reasoning and problem solving, disinhibition, perseveration, and poor planning and organization.

The neuropsychologist can assess the extent of cognitive impairments after hemorrhagic stroke. Outcome studies indicate those who survive hemorrhagic stroke do improve, with the maximal rate of improvement occurring in the first 6 months.[4] Patients can continue to experience cognitive recovery for longer intervals. Predictors of poor outcome include postsurgical vasospasm, increasing age, ACoA aneurysmal rupture, and systemic hypertension. Monitoring cognitive status is important, as cognitive status can indicate recovery variables. Popular cognitive screening instruments, such as the Mini-Mental State Examination, have age- and education-adjusted norms to facilitate interpretation of raw scores.[5,6]

The rehabilitation outcome of ICH survivors depends on the location of the hemorrhage and on bleeding characteristics such as the speed with which the hematoma was formed and its size. Survivors with deep, small ICH near midline structures often experience herniation and can have severe residual deficits.[2] For survivors with more superficial ICH, the outcome can be relatively good after blood has reabsorbed. The cognitive outcome from SAH is mixed and depends on the severity of brain injury and secondary complications. Individuals with relatively low scores on the Hunt-Hess scale might return to independent function. Similarly, persons with arteriovenous malformations may regain functional independence even after surgical resection. Serial neurobehavioral assessment uses a selective set of cognitive measures rather than a full neuropsychological test battery. Monitoring cognitive status can quantify changes in mental status that might signal hydrocephalus and toxic levels of anticonvulsant medication. Serial assessment can also identify residual deficits and suggest cognitive remediation using identified cognitive strengths to either facilitate recovery or to develop compensatory strategies to improve function. A full neuropsychological test battery can facilitate decisions about activities of daily living such as return to work and to driving.

The following case study demonstrates cognitive and functional recovery in a 19-year-old college student with a several-year history of headache who developed right hand numbness, agnosia, left-right confusion, and memory problems.[7] A computed tomography scan of the head revealed a large left occipitoparietal arteriovenous malformation with five feeding vessels. He underwent five embolization procedures. After the fourth, he was noted to have had an SAH, and subsequent to the fifth, he developed right homonymous hemianopsia. The arteriovenous malformation was resected in a left occipital partial lobectomy. There were two perioperative grand mal seizures. He remained seizure-free until a major motor seizure while playing a video game. Initial expressive aphasia improved. However, disconnection of the occipital cortex from the angular gyrus resulted in pure alexia. The student was motivated to return to college, graduate with a double major in communications and public relations, have extracurricular fun, and obtain a good job after graduation. He underwent extensive speech and occupational therapies for impaired word finding, reading, and math abilities. Early visual perceptual therapy included letter, number, and then shape cancellation tasks to increase reading speed. Visual comparisons and tangram puzzles were added to improve visual information processing. Letter-by-letter reading began with letter-recognition tasks that slowly increased to two-letter combinations. Compensatory strategies, such as placing work in the field of vision, tracking to the edge of the page, and using a memory book, were added. Later, he was encouraged to dictate information from television news shows into a tape recorder and to recall the main idea for texts. Visual motor exercises strengthened his dominant right hand. He was required to pick up increasingly smaller objects with his right hand. Integrated skills, including copying words while saying the letters and then the whole word out loud, appeared to facilitate letter-by-letter reading. Phonetic cues also helped word retrieval. When faced with word-finding difficulties, he would mouth letters of the alphabet until he identified the initial sound of the word he was seeking. Study skills and classroom adaptations were added as he readied for return to college. He was encouraged to search for the main idea, outline, obtain note takers, and request untimed multiple choice, not fill-in or essay, examinations. After one semester of auditing classes, he resumed college work with a laptop computer with an optical scanner and voice synthesizer. Serial neuropsychological assessment revealed the following cognitive recovery in the first year after his craniotomy. Screening for basic language functions indicated he had difficulty naming both a cross (e.g., "This is a red cross square.") and triangle. He was slightly more than one standard deviation below his peers on the Boston Naming Test. The capacity of working memory was significantly impaired relative to his age and education peers. He was able to boost his memory through the use of compensatory strategies learned in therapy and at school. However, when scores obtained 11/2 years after his craniotomy were compared with his own performances 4 months after surgery, he had experienced significant improvement in both visual-spatial memory and verbal memory together with moderate improvement on measures of attention, visual-spatial problem solving, reading recognition, abstract reasoning, and cognitive flexibility performances

Table 10.1 Functional Measurements Post Craniotomy

Measure	1 Mo	4 Mos	18 Mos
Trails A	—	29	29
Trails B	—	25	46
Seashore Rhythm	—	39	48
Speech Perception Test	—	36	52
Finger Tapping, Dominant	—	47	51
Finger Tapping, Nondominant	—	47	46
Verbal IQ	—	27	27
Performance IQ	—	25	32
Boston Naming Test	<1	19	37
Wechsler Memory Scale-Revised Memory Index	—	35	51

Raw scores transformed to T scores (mean = 50, SD = 10).

(Table 10.1). The subject had difficulty multiplying two numbers in his head. Drawings were well formed and placed. When reading out loud, he was slow, but accurate. He had to drop one major, but he did graduate as president of his college class. In addition, he was engaged and accepted at an internship. Although he was not formally assessed again, family reports indicated he continued to experience cognitive recovery and success in the world of work.

REFERENCES

1. D'Esposito M. Specific Stroke Syndromes. In: Mills VM, Cassity JW, Katz DI (eds). *Neurologic Rehabilitation: A Guide to Diagnosis, Prognosis, and Treatment Planning*. Malden, MA: Blackwell Science, 1997;59–103.
2. Chung C-S, Caplan LR. Neurovascular Disorders. In: Goetz CG, Pappert EJ (eds). *Textbook of Clinical Neurology*. Philadelphia: W.B. Saunders, 1999;907–932.
3. De Luca J, Diamond BJ. Aneurysm of the ACoA: A review of neuroanatomical and neuropsychological sequelae. *J Clin Exp Neuropsychol* 1995;17:100–121.
4. Brown GG, *et al*. The Effects of Cerebral Vascular Disease on Neuropsychological Functioning. In: Grant I, Adams KM (eds). *Neuropsychological Assessment of Neuropsychiatric Disorders, second edition*. New York: Oxford University Press, 1996;352.
5. Folstein MF, *et al*. Mini-Mental State: A practical method of grading the cognitive status of the patients for the clinician. *J Psychiatr Res* 1975;12:189–198.
6. Crum RA, *et al*. Population-based norms for the Mini-Mental State Examination by age and educational level. *JAMA* 1993;269:2386–2391.
7. Kaplan CP, *et al*. Cognitive improvement following partial left occipital lobectomy. *Proceedings of Applied Cognitive Remediation: 4th Training Seminar* 1997;17(Abstr.).

C

Treatment of Outpatients

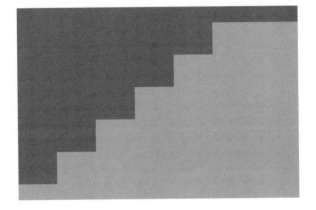

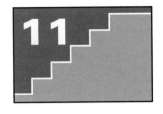

Musculoskeletal Manifestations of Hemorrhagic Stroke

Rene Cailliet

Once there has been a completed stroke, and neurologic residual impairment is manifested, the major portions of the limbs that manifest these impairments are the shoulder in the upper extremity and the foot-ankle in the lower. All aspects of the limbs, the hand and fingers and the hip and knee, are also important but are subservient to normal function of the shoulder and the foot-ankle.

Normal function of the extremities, upper and lower, is a complex neuromusculoskeletal activity that originates in the cerebral cortex and the midbrain, where basic pattern engrams are constructed. As the brain matures from birth, these "patterns" are modified by experience and later by repetition to perform the needed tasks of activities of daily living. New synapses are probably actually built (Figure 11.1).

Hemorrhagic stroke causes functional impairment of the musculoskeletal activities by interfering with the control by the cortex over the basic motor patterns that are encoded in the midbrain, the basal ganglia, and the cerebellum.

The loss of motor control of the cerebrum over the basic patterns in the upper extremity releases flexor patterns and in the lower extremity extensor patterns (Figure 11.2).

Before the impairments of either extremity are discussed, it is mandatory that normal function of these joints be considered.

UPPER EXTREMITIES

The upper extremity is a complex neuro-muscular-articular entity, with the role of the shoulder girdle being to place hand and fingers where the intended function is. Impairment of the shoulder girdle therefore impairs all arm, hand, and finger functions.

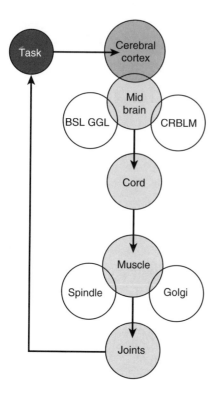

Figure 11.1 Neurophysiological sequence of muscular activities. The intended task initiates activities of the cerebral cortex and midbrain in patterns that are basic and modified with daily activity. The cerebellum (CRBLM) and basal ganglia (BSL GGL) also contain patterns. The activity of the muscle system is further modified by the spindle and Golgi systems. Sensory reaction modifies the performance, which reports back to the task.

Not only is upper extremity function impaired from a hemorrhagic stroke, but the resultant impaired function also causes pain, which presents a problem to both the patient and the therapy staff in an estimated 60% of patients who experience a stroke.[1]

Normal Shoulder Girdle Function

The term *shoulder girdle* is more appropriate, as the term *shoulder* comprises numerous articulations, all of which must function appropriately if the upper extremity also functions adequately (Figures 11.3 and 11.4). The numerous motions of the normal shoulder girdle are shown in Figure 11.5.

The major functional "joint" of the shoulder girdle can be considered to be the glenohumeral joint, as that is where the upper limb performs all of the motions depicted in Figure 11.5. This joint is complex (Figure 11.6).

The glenohumeral joint is considered to be an "incongruous" joint in which the adjacent bony curvatures are not symmetric; therefore, any movement is not merely rotation about a fixed axis of rotation, nor is the head fixed firmly within a deep concave joint (Figure 11.7).

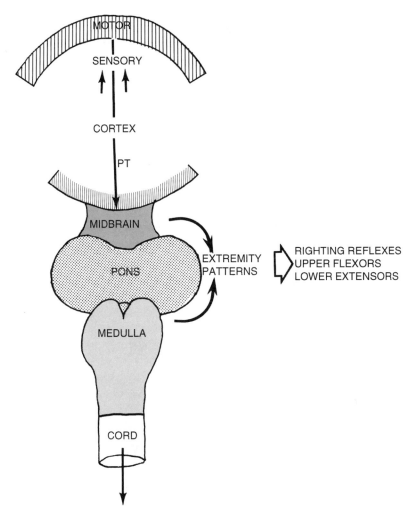

Figure 11.2 Release of basic patterns. When there is loss of motor and sensory control of the cortex over the basic patterns within the midbrain, pons, and medulla, basic patterns are released, which include flexor pattern of the upper extremity and extensor patterns of the lower extremities and the righting reflexes. Interruption from stroke occurs in the pyramidal tracts (PTs).

In the static position, the glenoid fossa, which is located at the distal end of the scapula, must be held at a specific angle to prevent the head of the humerus from gliding downward (Figures 11.8 and 11.9).

The head of the humerus is prevented from downward gliding by the superior portion of the capsule and the supraspinatus tendon (Figures 11.10 and 11.11).

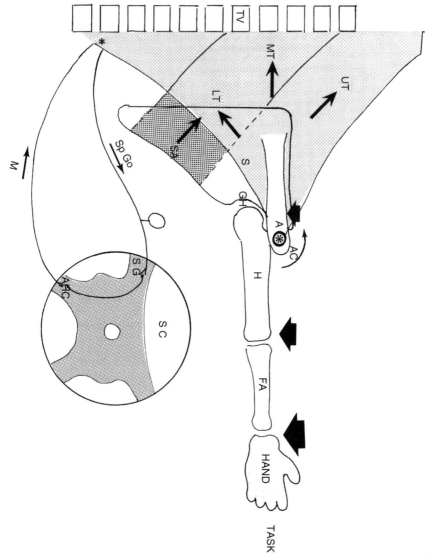

Figure 11.3 Complex neuromuscular trajectory of the upper extremity. In the trajectory phase, in which the shoulder places the hand in its functional position, the scapula (S) is activated by the trapezius muscle in its three divisions (upper [UT], middle [MT], and lower [LT]) and the serratus anterior (SA). The remainder of the extremity are the glenohumeral joint (GH), the acromium (A), acromioclavicular joint (AC), humerus (H), forearm (FA), and the hand. The asterisk is the axis of rotation of the glenohumeral joint. The neurologic motor control (M) of the scapula is from the sensory aspects of the spindle and Golgi systems (Sp Go) to the substantia gelatinosum (SG) that activates the anterior horn cells (AHC) supplying the afferent nerve fibers to the muscles. (SC = spinal cord; TV = thoracic vertebrae.)

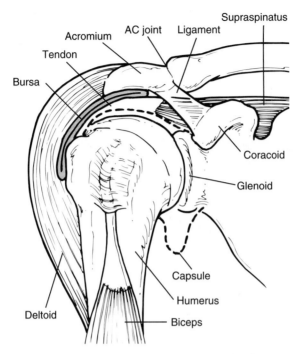

Figure 11.4 Shoulder girdle components. All of the components of the shoulder girdle are shown, indicating how numerous and closely packed they are. (AC joint = acromioclavicular joint.) (Reprinted with permission from Cailliet R. *Shoulder Pain, third edition*. Philadelphia: F.A. Davis, 1991;55.)

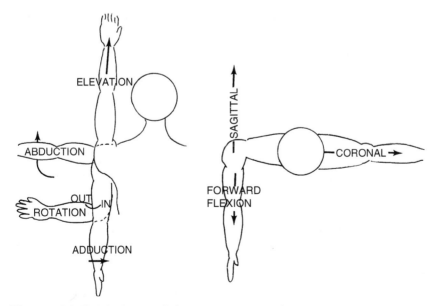

Figure 11.5 Motions of the upper extremity.

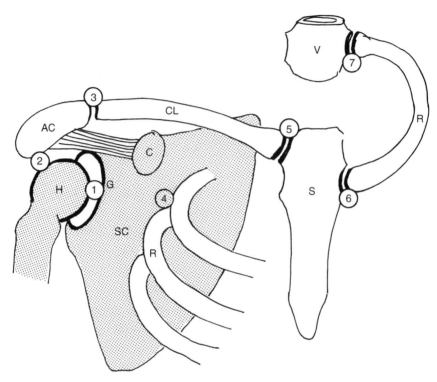

Figure 11.6 Components of the glenohumeral joint. The components of the shoulder girdle are (1) the glenohumeral joint (G); the
humeral head (H); (2) the suprahumeral joint; (3) the acromioclavicular joint; (4) the scapulocostal joint; (5) the sternoclavicular joint;
(6) the sternocostal joint; and (7) the costovertebral joint. (AC =
acromium; C = coracoid process; CL = clavicle; S = sternum; SC =
scapula; R = rib; V = vertebra.) (Adapted from Cailliet R. *Shoulder
Pain, third edition.* Philadelphia: F.A. Davis, 1991;2.)

The supraspinatus muscle, which is located in the supraspinatus
fossa of the scapula, has its tendon inserted on the greater tuberosity
of the humerus. It maintains its degree of isometric contraction via the
sensory impulses from its spindle system, which creates a local feedback system that modulates the velocity and force of contraction via
the gamma fibers and the alpha nerve fibers (Figure 11.12).

The intrafusal muscular modulators, the spindle system, and the
Golgi apparatus, which have been inferred, need clarification. The
intrafusal fibers of the spindle system reside within the extrafusal muscle fibers and essentially measure the different lengths of the muscle
(Figure 11.13).

In the spinal cord, there is interaction of the end organs of the spindle that determines the length and force needed to accomplish the

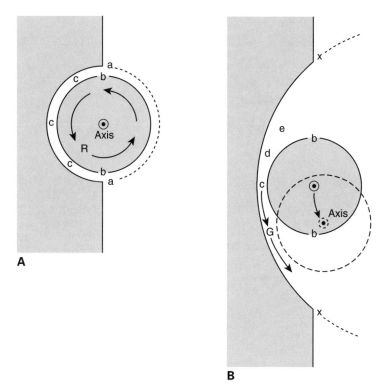

Figure 11.7 Congruity and incongruity. **A.** A congruous articula-
tion in which the male and female portions of the joint are symmetric and thus the distance between them is equal (c) at all points
(a–b). Movement is about a fixed axis of rotation (R). **B.** An incongruous joint in which the curvature of the female portion (x) differs
from the male portion (b). The joint spaces vary (c, d, e). Rotation
(*shaded* and *dotted*) requires a change of the axis of rotation, and
gravity (G) permits downward gliding.

intended task. The rate of change is a dynamic adaptation based on
sensory input (stereognosis). If stereognosis is lost as a result of stroke,
this mechanism is lost ("blinded").

The gamma afferent nerve fibers enter the cord from the spindle and
synapse to the anterior horn cells to initiate appropriate motor contraction of the extrafusal muscle fibers via alpha fibers.

The Golgi apparatus located in the tendons of the extrafusal muscle
fibers measure the force of contraction needed for the desired function.
Its afferent nerve fibers to the cord are via Ib fibers (Figure 11.14).

When the muscle is at rest, intrafusal and extrafusal fibers are of
equal length, and afferent impulses are minimal. On shortening or
lengthening in eccentric contraction of the muscle, the intrafusal (spindle) fibers also shorten, placing tension on the tendon. This coordinated

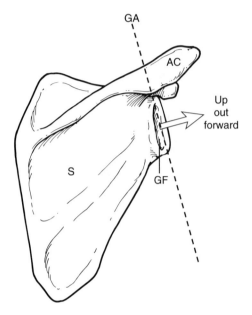

Figure 11.8 Angulation of the glenoid fossa (GF). The GF is located at the distal end of the scapula (S) under the acromium (AC). The glenoid angle (GA) faces the fossa upward, outward, and forward.

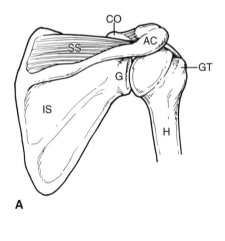

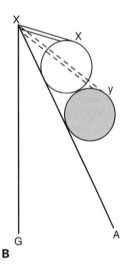

Figure 11.9 A. Shoulder girdle from the rear. **B.** Line of gravity (X–G). Elongation of the flaccid supraspinatus muscle (X–y) allows the humeral head (*shaded circle*) to descend. Decrease of the angle (X–A) also places strain on the supraspinatus muscle and superior capsule (not shown). (AC = acromium; CO = coracoid process; G = glenoid fossa; GT = greater tuberosity; H = humerus; IS = infraspinatus muscle; SS = supraspinatus muscle; X–X = support of the humerus from the supraspinatus muscle.)

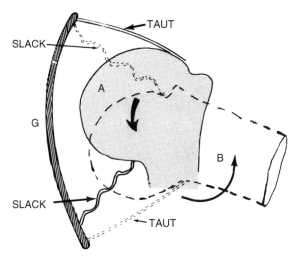

Figure 11.10 Capsular function of the glenohumeral joint. The shaded humeral head is held within the shallow glenoid fossa (G) by the taut superior capsule when the arm is dependent (A). The inferior aspect of the capsule is slack to permit abduction of the humerus (B). (Reprinted with permission from Cailliet R. *Shoulder Pain, third edition*. Philadelphia: F.A. Davis, 1991;268.)

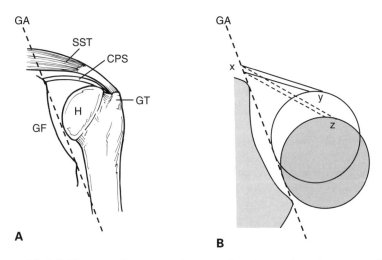

Figure 11.11 Supraspinatus action on the dependent humerus (H). **A.** The dependent humerus is prevented from downward gliding by the supraspinatus muscle (SST), which attaches on the greater tuberosity (GT) and the superior aspect of the capsule (CPS). The angle of the glenoid fossa (GF) is shown by the dotted line. **B.** Support of the SST tendon (x–y) is shown, which elongates (x–z) when the SST is flail. (GA = glenoid angle.)

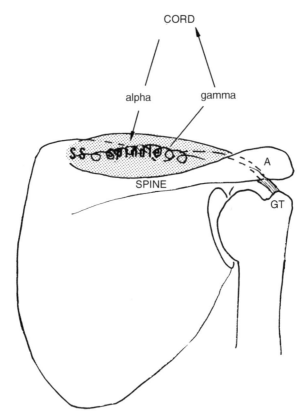

Figure 11.12 The supraspinatus muscle (SS). The SS contained within the supraspinatus fossa of the scapula has its tendon attached on the greater tuberosity (GT) of the humerus. The intrafusal spindle fiber notifies the cord via the gamma nerve fiber of the extent of contraction, which modulates the degree of contraction via the alpha fiber to the extrafusal muscle fibers of the muscle. (A = acromium.)

activity is imparted to the cord, where appropriate extrafusal activity ensues.

In the dependent arm (average weight, 15 lb), the supraspinatus muscle exerts just sufficient force to prevent subluxation from the glenoid fossa (see Figure 11.14). When active motion of the shoulder is initiated, there is active contraction of the supraspinatus muscle along with other rotator cuff muscles (Figure 11.15).

The bony glenoid fossa is shallow but is deepened with the labrum and further reinforced by the surrounding musculature (Figures 11.16 through 11.18).

Support of the normal dependent arm depends on an intact capsule and isometrically contracting rotator cuff muscles. The scapula must

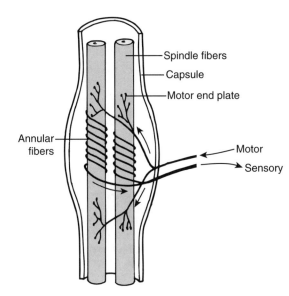

Figure 11.13 The spindle system. A simplified muscle spindle is depicted. Two intrafusal (spindle) fibers are enclosed within a connective tissue capsule. The sensory fibers become afferent to the cord. The "motor" fibers are "reset" in the spindle for the needed length and subsequent action.

also be sustained in the appropriate position to ensure the proper angulation of the glenoid fossa. This requires appropriate muscular contraction of all the scapular muscles. When the hemorrhagic stroke interferes with the control of these basic patterns, the "stroke shoulder" emerges with impaired and potential pain.

FLACCID STROKE PHASE

The initial phase of a stroke that may prove to be a transient ischemic attack or a completed stroke usually passes through a "flaccid stage," which may last for seconds, minutes, or a long period. The completed hemorrhagic stroke flaccid stage will probably last longer and make the patient vulnerable to Erb's palsy. This stage is the areflexive stage in which all reflexes are diminished or absent. During this stage, all voluntary movements are also lost, hence the term *flail*. Complete recovery may occur, or the patient may proceed to the spastic stage.

The shoulder in this flaccid stage undergoes specific changes that present concern for the future. The flaccid stage must be evaluated, reviewed frequently, and immediately managed, as its sequelae may be ominous for the functional pain-free future of the patient. The resultant traumatic brachial plexitis from traction that can occur during this flaccid stage is the reason for keeping the patient's arm and hand overhead in the bed and wheelchair positions.

The loss of reflex is combined with loss of intrinsic neurologic function. The upper motor neurons are "disconnected," and the intrinsic

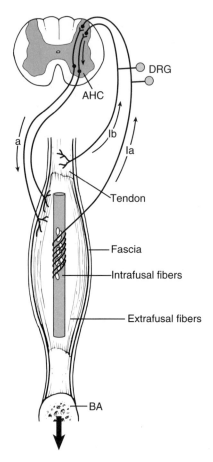

Figure 11.14 Intrafusal fiber connections. The intrafusal system is depicted. Two intra-fusal (spindle) fibers are encased within a connective tissue cap-sule. The sensory fiber from the spindle (Ia) is afferent to the cord ending in the gray matter. The Golgi apparatus within the tendon sends impulses via Ib fibers. The motor fiber that "resets" the spindle is not shown in the illustration. (a = motor fibers to extrafusal muscle fibers; AHC = anterior horn cells; BA = bony attachment; DRG = dorsal root ganglion.) (Reprinted with permission from Cailliet R. *Soft Tissue Pain and Disability, third edition.* Philadel-phia: F.A. Davis, 1997;63.)

neurologic "controllers," the spindle and Golgi systems, also become ineffectual. The musculature of the shoulder girdle essentially becomes flail, with no muscle contraction of any type.

The rotator cuff muscles of the glenohumeral joint become flail with excessive passive mobility and no motor control for kinetic action. Sensory and proprioceptive loss may also result. The significant loss is from loss of isometric contraction of the supraspinatus muscle (see Figure 11.12). As there is no isometric contraction of that muscle, the weight of the upper extremity is borne exclusively by the capsule, which has insufficient tone to maintain the humeral head within the glenoid fossa, hence allowing subluxation of the humerus from the glenoid fossa.

The muscles supporting the scapula are also areflexive and become flail, allowing the scapula to downward rotate from the weight of the arm, causing the angulation of the glenoid fossa to become vertical. This further causes a loss of depth of the fossa and the angulation of

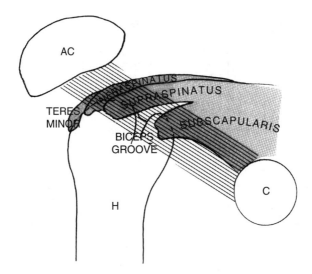

Figure 11.15 Rotator cuff muscles. The "rotator" cuff includes the supraspinatus, infraspinatus, teres minor, and the subscapularis muscles with a common tendon. (AC = acromium; C = coracoid process; H = humerus.)

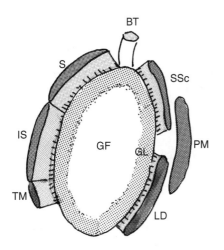

Figure 11.16 Downward movement of the head of the humerus within the glenoid fossa (GF). The humeral head glides downward within the GF from gravity and during active abduction or forward flexion of the arm. The surrounding muscles are as depicted in Figure 11.15. (BT = biceps tendon; GL = glenoid labrum; LD = latissimus dorsi; IS = infraspinatus muscle; PM = pectoralis major-minor; S = supraspinatus muscle; SSc = subscapularis muscle; TM = teres minor.)

the superior portion of the capsule that "seats" the head of the humerus.

The loss of righting reflexes as well as proprioceptive stimulation of the vertebral paraspinous muscles cause a "functional" scoliosis, with lateral curvature to the affected side. This causes further downward rotation of the scapula and further change in the vertical angulation of the glenoid fossa (Figure 11.19).

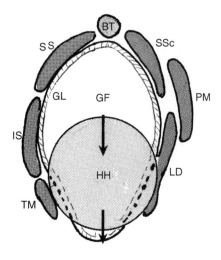

Figure 11.17 Downward movement of the humeral head (HH) within the glenoid fossa (GF). The HH glides downward within the GF from gravity during active abduction or forward flexion of the arm. The surrounding muscles are as depicted in Figure 11.15. (BT = biceps tendon; GL = glenoid labrum; IS = infraspinatus muscle; LD = latissimus dorsi; PM = pectoralis major-minor; SS = supraspinatus muscle; SSc = subscapularis muscle; TM = teres minor.)

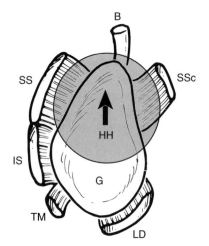

Figure 11.18 Elevation of the humeral head (HH). Any active or passive movement of the HH superiorly is contained within the glenoid fossa (G) by the biceps tendon (B) and all of the muscles located superiorly: the supraspinatus (SS) and subscapularis (SSc) muscles. (IS = infraspinatus; LD = latissimus dorsi; TM = teres minor.)

All three parts of the deltoid muscle that act to maintain the head of the humerus within the suprahumeral space are also ineffective. The three parts of the deltoid function in a different manner dependent on their lines of pull and have a differential contraction rate through the biofeedback system initiated by sensory afferent fibers from the capsule of the glenohumeral joint. The anterior portion of the deltoid muscle is not an abductor but requires supraspinatus contraction to be an abductor and forward flexor. The loss of the supraspinatus muscle obviously does not substitute deltoid function in preventing subluxation, but it partially antagonizes deltoid function in its new spatial orientation (Figure 11.20).

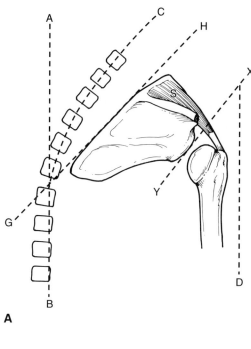

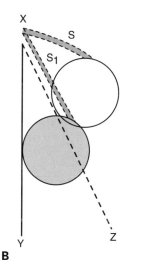

Figure 11.19
Functional scoliosis.
A. The vertebral column (thoracic; A–B) bends toward the side of the stroke (B–C), causing the downward rotation of the scapula (G–H) and, hence, changes the angulation of the glenoid fossa (Y–X). The humerus becomes abducted (D). The supraspinatus muscle (S) normally would prevent downward movement of the humerus.
B. The glenoid angle (X–Z) is changed, and the supraspinatus muscle tendon is now passively elongated (S_1) and unable to prevent subluxation (*shaded ball*).

It becomes apparent that the entire musculature of the shoulder girdle becomes involved in the flaccid stage of the stroke, and each component muscle must be addressed.

There are proprioceptor end organs within joint capsules that initiate muscular action to stabilize the joint. These are not functional in the flaccid stroke phase[2–4] and, thus, from any passive stretch of the

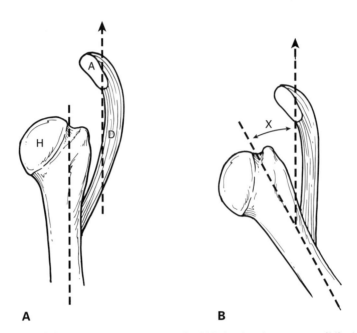

A   **B**

Figure 11.20 Deltoid function. **A.** With the humerus (H) dependent, the deltoid muscle (D) attaches vertically from the acromium
(A) to the upper portion of the humerus and elevates (*arrow*) the
humerus into the suprahumeral joint area. **B.** With the humerus
abducted (X) from rotator cuff action, the deltoid is now able to
contract and further abduct the humerus (see text for details).

capsules and tendons there may occur a separation of the joint, as there
occurs no reflex contraction of the muscles, which are, at this phase,
totally flaccid.

Clinical Aspect

In the patient with completed stroke, the shoulder presents possible
subluxation that can be noted by an increased space between the
acromium and the humeral head (as compared to the contralateral
side). This is palpably noted and can be verified by appropriate x-rays
with the patient erect to cause the arm to be dependent.

There is no active motion of the arm in abduction or forward or
backward flexion and no external rotation. These actions depend on
contraction of the rotator cuff muscles. A lateral scoliosis can be noted
when the patient is placed and supported in the seated or standing
erect position. Scapular elevation or protraction, or both, is limited if
even possible.

Pain is not necessarily present as a sign of subluxation, although pain is present in 60% of stroke patients within 2–3 months as the stroke persists or progresses into the spastic or synergic phase.

Treatment

Management of the flaccid phase of the hemiplegic shoulder is to passively and actively prevent the effects of gravity and enhance muscular contraction of the supraspinatus muscle by numerous means. Use of a sling has been proven to be ineffectual and even detrimental as reviewed by the literature and is therefore not discussed.

The patient can be taught and assisted to roll in the prone or supine position on the affected side. In the seated position, the extended arm, with palm to the surface of the furniture on which the patient is seated, supports the body against challenges to being upright and forces the head of the humerus superiorly against the acromium and the coracohumeral ligament.

Stimulation of the supraspinatus muscle can be initiated by electrical stimulation and repeated numerous times daily, brushing and tapping the muscle until there is evidence of some active contraction or some spasticity. Vibration has been advocated as stimulating the spindle proprioceptive mechanism and is worth implementing into the treatment protocol.[5]

SPASTIC HEMIPLEGIC SHOULDER

The completed stroke usually progresses into the spastic phase in which many or all of the muscles of the shoulder girdle undergo spasticity. As stated, the midbrain, which contains the basic patterns, is now in control, and the flexor patterns predominate.

Before discussing the spastic shoulder, the kinetic normal shoulder must be discussed. As the intent of the upper extremity function is initiated to place the hand in its functional position, the shoulder becomes "kinetic." The shoulder girdle that has been maintained as a supportive proximal structure holding the dependent arm now becomes active to place the hand in its functional site. The spastic shoulder nearly always is accompanied by dynamic sensory "blindness" (stereognosis, etc.) with the arm receiving little feedback as it moves passively or actively through space.

On the total upper extremity function becoming kinetic, all of the muscles of the glenohumeral joint become active in some type of contraction. The numerous types of muscle contraction are stated as being

Concentric: Contractions that produce motion through their shortening. The internal force exceeds the external force of resistance.

Eccentric: Contraction occurs as the shortened muscle length continues to maintain tension.

Isometric: Contraction has no external movement, as the external resistance equals the internal force.

Isotonic: Internal contraction equals the external resistance force with no resultant movement.

Anisotonic: Contraction occurs during motion with either concentric (positive work) or eccentric (negative work) contraction.

Many motions require combined types of contraction, and this must be ascertained from a competent evaluation.

The scapular and glenohumeral muscles that have been contracting isometrically now contract isokinetically to produce the desired motion with appropriate force and speed as determined by the intended arm-hand motion. The force and speed are monitored at the spindle and Golgi systems and are monitored by the upper motor neurons in specified motor patterns.

The supraspinatus muscle actively contracts to abduct and forward flex the humerus in the direction needed. This muscle is an abductor-flexor as well as an external rotator, with the action(s) determined by which motions of the patterns are needed (Figure 11.21).

During this glenohumeral motion, the scapula remains stable as the scapular muscles contract isotonically with appropriate force to support the arm that is now deviating from the vertical plane.

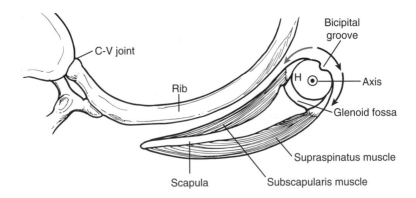

Figure 11.21 Motions of the supraspinatus muscle. Viewed superiorly, the supraspinatus muscle externally rotates about the axis within the humerus (H), and the subscapularis internally rotates the humerus. (C-V = costovertebral joint.) (Reprinted with permission from Cailliet R. *Shoulder Pain, third edition*. Philadelphia: F.A. Davis, 1991;33.)

The external rotation force is not yet significantly expended, as that motion may not yet be needed in the total upper extremity pattern. The internal rotators, which are powerful due to their structure angle of insertion giving mechanical advantage, in this action have actively suppressed. The internal rotators are the subscapularis muscle of the rotator cuff (Figure 11.22), the latissimus dorsi muscle, and the pectoralis muscles (Figure 11.23).

As the arm abducts and forward flexes, all the muscles contract with increased force as the arm and hand move from the center of gravity and antagonistic muscles reciprocally relax. As the humerus abducts and flexes, the scapula tends to move in what is termed the *scapulohumeral rhythm*. From vertical alignment of the dependent arm, as the humerus abducts and elevates, the scapula, when it moves, moves in a 2 to 1 ratio: 2 of the humerus and 1 of the scapula (Figure 11.24).

As the humerus abducts or forward flexes, the greater tuberosity of the humerus impinges on the acromium and the coracohumeral ligament at 90 degrees, preventing further elevation. The humerus impinges at 60 degrees abduction with the humerus internally rotated, but external rotation permits abduction to 120 degrees as with this

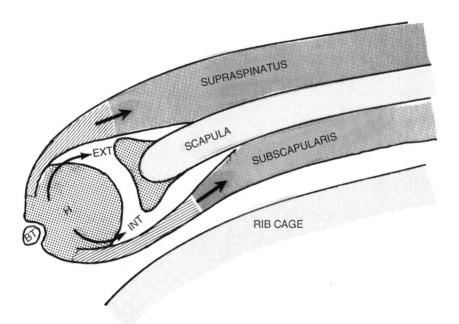

Figure 11.22 Subscapularis muscle. Viewed from above, the rotation action on the humerus (H) of the supraspinatus muscle is external rotation (EXT) and of the subscapularis muscle is internal rotation (INT). (BT = biceps tendon.)

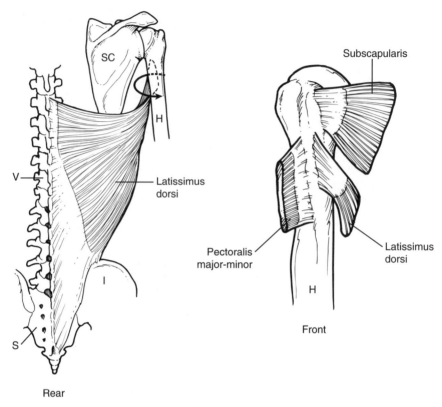

SC

H

V

Latissimus
dorsi

I

S

Rear

Subscapularis

Pectoralis
major-minor

Latissimus
dorsi

H

Front

Figure 11.23 Latissimus dorsi, subscapularis, and pectoralis muscle attachments. Rear view: The attachments on the humerus (H) of the latissimus dorsi externally rotate the humerus (*dotted arrow*). Front view: The pectoralis major-minor, subscapularis, and latissimus dorsi muscles are shown attaching to the humerus. (I = ilium; S = sacrum; SC = scapula; V = vertebrae.)

rotation the greater tuberosity moves behind the coracohumeral ligament and the acromium (Figure 11.25).

It is apparent that for normal upper limb movement all aspects of the scapula and the humerus must function in a coordinated action, and the antagonist muscles must relax appropriately. These antagonistic muscles to the serratus anterior include the levator scapulae and the rhomboid muscles, which are not strong and have a low mechanical advantage (Figure 11.26).

The paraspinous muscles must also be incorporated in the scapulohumeral action, as the contralateral muscles must contract to balance the thoracic spine and prevent functional scoliosis from the weight of the arm (see Figure 11.23). These muscles are activated by the righting reflexes contained within the midbrain.

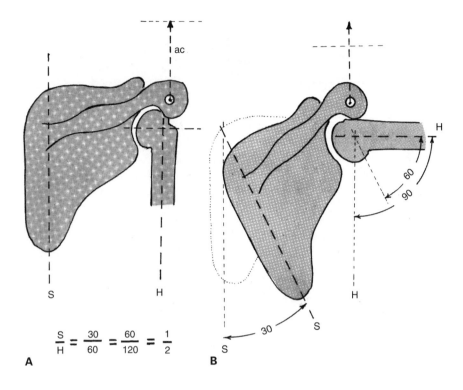

$$\frac{S}{H} = \frac{30}{60} = \frac{60}{120} = \frac{1}{2}$$

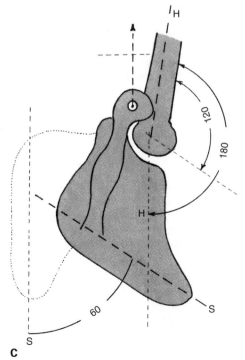

Figure 11.24
Scapulohumeral rhythm.
The scapulohumeral rhythm
(S/H) is shown. **A.** Arm is
dependent, and the scapula
(S) and humerus (H) are
parallel. **B.** Humerus is
abducted to 90 degrees: 60
at the glenohumeral joint
and 30 at the scapulotho-
racic joint. **C.** Arm is totally
elevated (180 degrees): 60
at the scapula and 120 at
the glenohumeral joint.
(ac = acromium.)

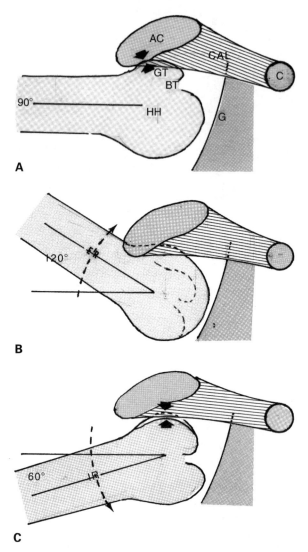

Figure 11.25 Effect of humerus rotation on arm elevation. **A.** Impingement of the greater tuberosity (GT) of the head of the humerus (HH) on the acromium (AC), with the coracoacromial ligament (CAL) at 90 degrees. **B.** The humerus is externally rotated (ER). **C.** With the humerus internally rotated (IR), impingement occurs at 60 degrees. (BT = biceps tendon; C = coracoid process; G = glenoid fossa.)

The completed stroke impairs this coordinated action of the shoulder girdle. Some muscles eccentrically contract and some relax. The biofeedback is also impaired, therefore impairing this intricate function.

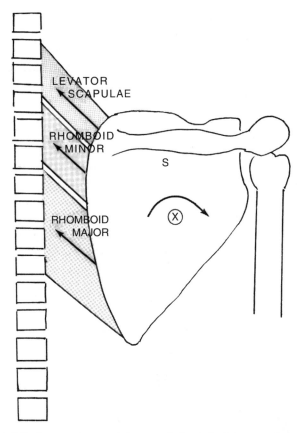

Figure 11.26 Levator scapulae and rhomboid muscles are shown and by their origin and insertion angle cause the scapula (S) to downward rotate about the axis (X). (Reprinted with permission from Cailliet R. *The Functional Anatomy of the Musculoskeletal System: Illustrated.* Tokyo: Ishiyaku Publishers, 1990.)

As has been stated, the supraspinatus muscle initially becomes flail and unable to support the humeral head within the glenoid fossa. Now with the kinetic phase being initiated, the flexor synergy, or any part, becomes activated. The abductor and flexor muscles are not in this synergy and thus are ineffectual to abduct, forward flex, and externally rotate the humerus. The internal rotators and the subscapularis, pectoralis, and latissimus dorsi muscles, being in the now-uncontrolled flexor pattern, adduct and internally rotate the arm and downward rotate the glenoid fossa of the scapula. The levator scapula and rhomboid muscles contract unopposed, further depressing the scapula. The spastic ipsilateral paraspinous muscles and inactive contralateral paraspinous muscles now permit lateral scoliosis. All these actions on the scapula change the angulation of the glenoid fossa, permitting downward motion of the humeral head, furthering the subluxation and imposing the gravity effect on the capsule.

BICEPS FUNCTION

The biceps tendon function has not been discussed and therefore its role in the hemiparetic shoulder not implicated. The biceps normally acts "passively" to depress the head of the humerus during abduction and forward flexion. The head of the humerus passes over the biceps tendon, which is in the biceps fossa. The biceps tendon does not "actively" pass over the biceps groove, but its passive contraction from biceps contraction tenses the tendon, making it more efficient (Figure 11.27). In the spastic hemiparetic shoulder, the biceps muscle also becomes spastic and functionally "shortens" the biceps tendon, caus-

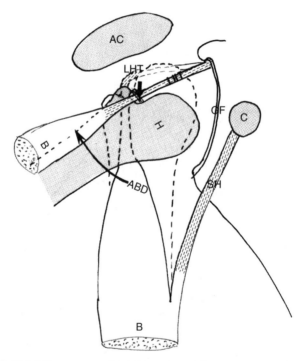

Figure 11.27 Biceps tendon function. The dependent arm is the dotted figure showing the biceps tendon (LHT) crossing at a right angle. As the arm abducts (ABD), the humeral head (H) descends on the glenoid fossa (GF). The biceps (B), with its long head tendon, depresses the humerus (*small arrow*). The short head of the biceps (SH) attaches to the coracoid process (C), but the coracoid process is not involved in the abduction process. (AC = acromium.)

ing it to increase downward movement of the head of the humerus leading to further subluxation.

The hemiparetic shoulder action is now fully implemented. Normal arm function placing the hand where it is needed for the intended action is no longer possible.

CLINICAL EVALUATION

The patient with hemorrhagic stroke presents the classic hemiparetic shoulder girdle: The arm is adducted and internally rotated, the scapula droops, the unaffected arm lies closer to the vertebrae with the inferior angle adducted ("retracted"), and the vertebral border is pulled away from the rib cage. The increased tonus in the muscles makes it difficult to actively or passively mobilize in any direction.

Because the scapula rotates downward, causing the glenoid fossa to be vertical, the arm appears to be in a relatively abducted orientation as the arm remains against the body. This causes the capsule (superior aspect) not to be taut, allowing the head of the humerus to further sublux downward.

As the impairment progresses, there is evident atrophy of the supraspinatus, infraspinatus, and posterior portion of the deltoid muscles. The separation of the humerus from the capsule is visible and palpable.

TREATMENT OBJECTIVES

The position of the glenohumeral joint must be returned to its locking mechanism with restoration of the normal angle of the glenoid fossa, which means returning the scapula to its normal position. To do this means decreasing the spasticity of all the scapular muscles that are placing it in its hemiplegic position. The restored position must be maintained day and night. Vibration of these spastic muscles has been shown to decrease the spasticity allegedly from influencing the spindle system. The "weak" paretic muscles must be stimulated to regain strength and restore reciprocal relaxation of the antagonistic muscles. This increased contractile strengthening may be attempted by electrical stimulation, tapping, stroking, and using the numerous techniques of "muscle re-education."

Restoration of function of the hand, fingers, and wrist after a completed stroke must take into consideration the neurologic aspect of the distal portion of the upper extremity. The flexor synergy that occurs as compared to the extensor synergy of the lower extremity has the following components: the shoulder girdle has been addressed, and the elbow flexes, the forearm pronates, the wrist flexes, the fingers flex and adduct, and the thumb flexes and adducts in conjunction with internal rotation of the shoulder.

Although flexor synergy is predominant occasionally, an extensor synergy of the upper extremity can occur in which the elbow extends with pronation of the forearm, the wrist extends somewhat, the fingers flex with adduction, and the thumb adducts in flexion. It is apparent that in extensor synergy only the elbow and forearm vary from the flexor synergy.

PAINFUL SHOULDER

The pathogenesis of pain occurring in the hemiparetic shoulder are all the factors that cause pain in the normal mechanically injured shoulder. This includes tendonitis, bursitis, partial tear of the rotator cuff, complete tear of the rotator cuff, adhesive capsulitis (the "frozen shoulder"), and reflex sympathetic dystrophy, currently termed *complex regional pain syndrome*,[6] which is discussed further in Chapter 12.

REFERENCES

1. Davis PJ. *Shoulder Problems Associated with Hemiplegia. "Steps to Follow Guide to the Treatment of Adult Hemiplegia."* New York: Springer-Verlag, 1985;206–240.
2. Clark FJ, *et al*. Proprioception with the proximal interphalangeal joint of the index finger. *Brain* 1986;19:1195–1208.
3. Johnsson H. Role of knee ligaments in proprioception and regulation of muscle stiffness. *J Electromyogr Kinesiol* 1991;1:158–179.
4. Johansson H, *et al*. Receptors in the knee joint ligaments and their role in the biomechanics of the joint. *Crit Rev Biomed Eng* 1991;18:341–368.
5. Brumagne S, *et al*. The role of paraspinous muscle spindles in lumbosacral position sense in individuals with and without low back pain. *Spine* 2000; 25:989–994.
6. Cailliet R. *Shoulder Pain, third edition*. Philadelphia: F.A. Davis, 1991.

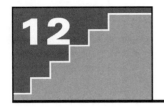

12 Complex Regional Pain Syndrome

Rene Cailliet

One of the ominous causes of painful shoulder is shoulder-hand-finger syndrome, which is a variant of complex regional pain syndrome (CRPS). The relationship is arbitrary, because CRPS is a neurologic syndrome of the autonomic nervous system, and shoulder-hand syndrome is a secondary complication of painful hemiplegic shoulder, which is considered to be reflex sympathetic dystrophy (RSD), as it has responded to sympathetic nerve blocks and has many manifestations of CRPS.

The shoulder-hand-finger syndrome occurs in an estimated 12.5% of post-hemiplegic patients with painful shoulders.[1] The relationship to the shoulder is that most patients who develop the RSD syndrome have a residual hemiplegic shoulder that is dependent and unable to be elevated above heart level. These patients also have a paretic hand that remains flexed with inability to extend wrist and fingers (Figure 12.1), but there are other pathoanatomic factors that occur.

This syndrome can be over- or underdiagnosed in any painful shoulder from whatever cause. What must be ascertained is the presence of objective neurovascular changes that are noted rather than merely relying on symptomatology.

This syndrome usually has its onset between the first and third month after the onset of stroke. In the medical literature, the onset of shoulder-hand syndrome has time factors as shown in Table 12.1.[2,3]

The patient's hand suddenly becomes swollen, with marked limitation of range of motion. Pain, at first, is not prominent, if at all present, and therefore the swollen hand is often ignored. In the 60–80% of patients who develop a painful shoulder after a hemorrhagic stroke, the hand swelling painlessly appears in only 12.5% of patients.

The shoulder-hand syndrome was initially considered a variant of RSD when, in 1958, the symptoms were relieved by a sympathetic stellate nerve block, implicating the autonomic nervous system.[4] These blocks relieved the hand findings but had no effect on the symptoms and findings of the shoulder. There were few well-controlled and

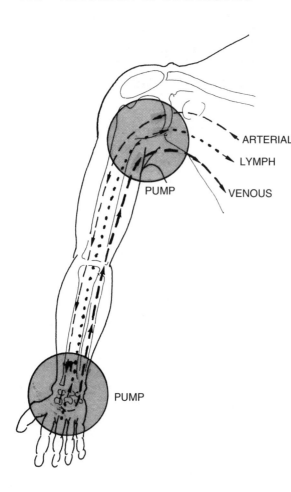

ARTERIAL

LYMPH

PUMP

VENOUS

PUMP

Figure 12.1
Shoulder and hand
"pumps." The
shoulder action
pumps arterial and
venous blood as
well as lymph. The
hand also "pumps"
arterial and venous
blood and lymph
toward the heart.
(Reprinted with
permission from
Cailliet R. *The
Shoulder in Hemi-
plegia.* Philadel-
phia: F.A. Davis,
1980;108.)

blinded studies, therefore leading to empirical treatments. Oral steroids
did have a beneficial effect when combined with physical therapeutic
modalities.[1]

It is safe to this point in time to say that the cause of CRPS and hence
the shoulder-hand syndrome remains unclear. Its objective diagnosis

Table 12.1 Time to Onset of Shoulder-Hand Syndrome

Months	Percentage of Patients
0–1	0
1–2	28
2–3	37
3–4	16
4–5	17
5–6	2

also remains unclear. Merely the dependency of the hand cannot be the etiology, as many patients who sustain this hand dependency do not have residual symptoms of the syndrome, but it remains a factor that must be addressed.

The hand, which remains in the palmar flexed position, undergoes venous obstruction. This has been verified by contrast medium injected into the hand veins and x-rayed in neutral and forcefully flexed positions. The wrist position and not the spasticity of the upper extremity muscles must be considered a causative factor, as often there is no significant spasticity at this stage of the syndrome and in fact the extremity may still be in the flaccid stage.

The presence of Raynaud's vasculitis, systemic lupus erythematosus, and other neurovascular entities must be considered and differentiated.

STAGES

The early stage of shoulder-hand syndrome is acute swelling of the hand, usually on the dorsum of the fingers where the creases of the fingers at the metacarpal phalangeal and proximal interphalangeal joints is initially noted. The original edema is soft and can be indented by pressure from the examiner. The normally visible extensor tendons are no longer seen. The edema is localized and ends just proximal to the wrist.

The venous supply of the hand is on the dorsum, and lymph that exudes from obstructed veins fills the space between the extensor tendons and the bones, initially being responsible for the limited flexion (Figure 12.2).

The collateral ligaments of the metacarpal-phalangeal joint normally are slack when the fingers are extended to their physiologic limits to permit full flexion of that joint (Figure 12.3).

The edema under the extensor tendon also extends under the collateral ligaments, thus extending them before there is full flexion of the joint and maintaining some flexion.[5] The edema contains protein that converts into a cobweb-like scar tissue that adheres the tendons to the joint capsules. As gradual adhesive limitation of joint movement occurs, the nutrition to the cartilage is diminished, causing atrophic degenerative changes.

Hyperesthesia appears early in the onset of CRPS. In fact, it may be the original symptom and sign that indicates its advent. As the shoulder-hand (CRPS) syndrome progresses, the skin changes to a pink color, indicating vasomotor dilation. This is particularly noted when the hand is held dependent for prolonged periods and diminishes when elevated. The skin feels warm and is moist (hyperhydrosis). Joint range

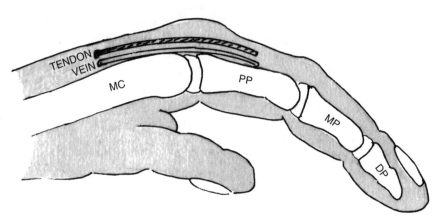

Figure 12.2 Venous supply to the hand. The veins are on the dorsum of the hand, and the edema that forms is under the extensor tendons as well as over them. (DP = dorsalis pedis; MC = metacarpal; MP = metaphalangeal; PP = proximal phalanx.)

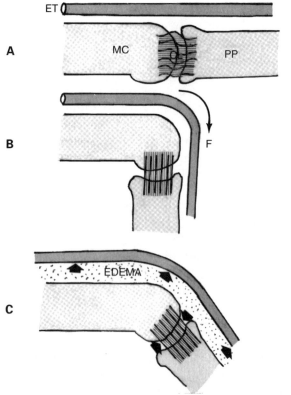

Figure 12.3 Collateral ligaments of the metacarpal-phalangeal joints. **A.** With the joint extended, the collateral ligaments are slack and become taut at full flexion (F) **(B)**. **C.** In the edematous hand, the fluid migrates between these collateral ligaments and prevents full extension of the ligaments and thus decreased flexion of the finger. (ET = extensor tendon; MC = metacarpal; PP = proximal phalanx.)

of motion, passive and active, is initially noted in supination of the wrist and forearm and metacarpal-phalangeal flexion. Gradually, the limitation occurs in distal phalangeal flexion and abduction of the fingers (Figures 12.4 and 12.5).

In evaluating this impaired joint function, it must be noted that the metacarpal-phalangeal joint is an incongruous joint and that flexion is not around a fixed axis but rather is a downward glide that precedes flexion (Figure 12.6). This is important in evaluating range-of-motion testing and, ultimately, in treatment.

LATER STAGES OF
HAND-SHOULDER SYNDROME

All the symptoms progress in the hand that is not treated appropriately and early in hand-shoulder syndrome. Allodynia (excessive sensitivity to what is normal, accepted, tactile sensation) makes normal function difficult and treatment using manual contact impossible. No abnormalities are noted on electromyography or nerve conduction time studies.

The ligaments gradually become ossified, the joint cartilages undergo disuse atrophy, the joint capsules thicken, the tendons and the joint capsules adhere to each other, and the bone undergoes osteoporosis. In the final stage (III), the hand is totally fixed in a flexed position with

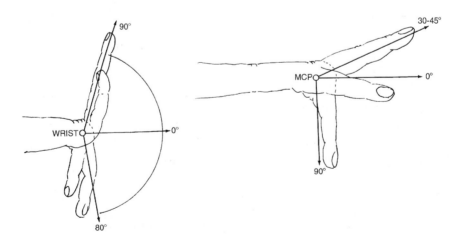

Figure 12.4 Normal range of motion in the hand. The normal joint ranges of motion of the wrist and metacarpal-phalangeal (MCP) joints are noted. (Reprinted with permission from Cailliet R. *Hand Pain and Impairment, fourth edition.* Philadelphia: F.A. Davis, 1994;12.)

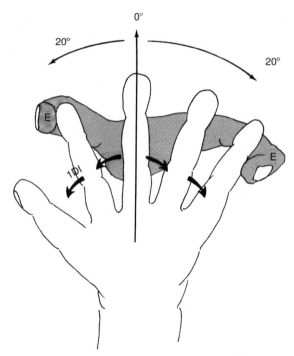

Figure 12.5 Abduction of the fingers. The fingers abduct about the middle finger (0) with the other fingers 20 degrees from the midline. (1DI = first digit; E = examiner.) (Reprinted with permission from Cailliet R. *Hand Pain and Impairment, fourth edition.* Philadelphia: F.A. Davis, 1994;53.)

no active or passive motion possible and, therefore, functionless. The allodynia gradually diminishes.

CHARACTERISTIC PAIN

CRPS, initially termed *RSD*, is a symptom complex characterized by vasomotor instability, hyperesthesia, and pain, usually of a "burning" quality. Kosin[6] proposed the following four clinical criteria for the diagnosis of RSD: (1) pain in an extremity, (2) vasomotor instability, (3) edema of the extremity, and (4) dystrophic skin changes.

More recently, the standards published in 1994[7] are being questioned as being based on clinical findings with no pathoanatomic basis, leading to under- and overdiagnosis of shoulder-hand syndrome. The proposed criteria are[8]

1. Continuing pain that is disproportionate to any inciting event.

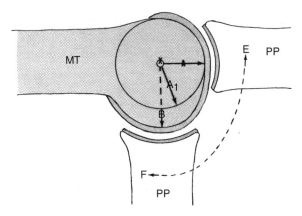

Figure 12.6 Motion of the metacarpal-phalangeal joint. The meta-carpal head (MT) is ovoid (X–B) rather than round (X–A). Extension (E) of the proximal phalanx (PP) is free, but flexion (F) is downward flexion then rotation about the metacarpal head. (A_1 = alpha$_1$ receptor.) (Reprinted with permission from Cailliet R. *Hand Pain and Impairment, fourth edition.* Philadelphia: F.A. Davis, 1994;33.)

2. Must report at least one symptom in each of the four following categories:
   a. *Sensory*: Reports of hyperesthesia
   b. *Vasomotor*: Reports of temperature asymmetry or skin color changes, or both, and/or skin color asymmetry
   c. *Sudomotor/edema*: Reports of edema or sweating changes, or both, and/or sweating symmetry
   d. *Motor/trophic*: Reports of decreased range of motion or motor dysfunction (weakness, tremor, dystonia), or both, and/or trophic changes (hair, nails, skin)
3. Must display at least one sign in two or more of the following categories:
   a. *Sensory*: Evidence of hyperalgesia (to pin prick) or allodynia (to light touch), or both
   b. *Vasomotor*: Evidence of temperature asymmetry or skin color changes, or both, and/or asymmetry
   c. *Sudomotor/edema*: Evidence of edema or sweating changes, or both, and/or sweating asymmetry
   d. *Motor/trophic*: Evidence of decreased range of motion or motor dysfunction (weakness, tremor, dystonia), or both, and/or trophic changes of the hair, nails, and skin

Alpha-adrenoceptors, particularly alpha$_1$-adrenoceptors, have been implicated in the development of "sympathetic" pain.[7,8] In RSD (now considered CRPS), it is postulated that there is "hypo" activity of the sympathetic nervous system that permits "hyper" activity of the alpha-adrenoreceptors to norepinephrine in blood vessels and their nociceptive end organs (Figure 12.7).[7]

Drummond et al.[9] found lower levels of noradrenaline in the limb affected with RSD. This increased responsiveness of alpha-adrenocep-tors and mechanoreceptors may explain the allodynia in RSD. Relief of allodynia by guanethidine injections, which block alpha-adrenogenic impulses, confirms the adrenogenic concept.[10] All of these findings may lead to a more effective treatment of RSD.

Sympathetic pain, originally refuted, is now considered possible due to the plasticity of the central nervous system.[9,11,12] The pain is triggered by stimulation of neurovascular thermoreceptor C fibers sensitized to norepinephrine. Pain is considered a disturbance of

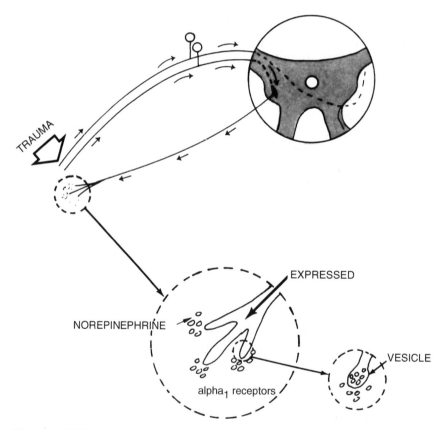

Figure 12.7 Alpha₁-receptor activity in reflex sympathetic dystro-phy. Trauma liberates release of autonomic impulses by stimulation of the lateral horn cells, which stimulate the sympathetic ganglia. These impulses liberate norepinephrine, which in turn stimulates the alpha₁-receptors. See text for details. (Reprinted with permis-sion from Cailliet R. *Pain: Mechanisms and Management.* Philadel-phia: F.A. Davis, 1993;47.)

microcirculation generated by small C fibers in the wall of the arterioles.[12–14] These are not large enough to be detected by nerve conduction studies. These afferent pain fibers terminate in the contralateral parietal sensory cortex, and in CRPS, the polysynaptic sensory fibers terminate bilaterally in the limbic system.[15] This is considered to explain the symptoms of insomnia, irritability, and depression in CRPS.

The etiology of CRPS includes trauma, which is usually minor and usually a repetitive stress injury. The selective injury to C fibers in the absence of trauma to the myelinated somatic nerve fibers leave the smaller C fibers uninhibited and lead to hypersensitivity of the circulatory norepinephrine, increasing C-fiber firing and sensitization of the spinal cord.[16,17]

CRPS must be recognized early when there is instantaneous edema immediately after a minor trauma to an extremity. This is also true in the post-stroke patient without trauma. Asymmetric excessive sweating (hyperhydrosis) is also a major warning sign.[18]

Application of ice, which is commonly applied in this condition, exaggerates vasoconstriction and may damage the myelinated nerve fibers if used excessively and for prolonged periods. This is the reason for using massage therapy and moist heat along with nerve blocks rather than ice.

CONFIRMATORY TESTS IN DIAGNOSIS

Once the symptoms suggest CRPS, the following tests have been used to confirm the diagnosis:

- Scintigraphic triphasic bone scanning is positive in approximately 55% of cases, and thus is not above random statistical yield.
- Diagnostic nerve blocks: Phentolamine and guanethidine are usually diagnostic in early cases but gradually lose their sensitivity.
- Electromyographic and nerve conduction time studies show no abnormality in CRPS, as the nerves involved are unmyelinated somatic or autonomic.
- Computed tomography and magnetic resonance imaging do not detect damage of the microscopic nerve fibers in the walls of blood vessels. They become informative with early osteoporosis.
- The quantitative sudomotor axon reflex that evaluates the cholinergic sudomotor function of the autonomic nervous system does not address the norepinephrine dysfunction.[19]
- Infrared thermal imaging has limited application and can only identify areas of damage and cannot determine the time factors as too old, new, or pre-existing.[20]

- Laser Doppler flow study is sensitive for the study of capillary circulation.[21]

STAGES

Before discussing treatment, the stages of CRPS in their temporal course should be clarified.

Stage I: Sympathetic dysfunction with thermatomal distribution (not dermatomal); mostly subjective.
Stage II: Dystrophy emerges with edema, hyperhydrosis, and neurovascular instability evident by skin color changes. There may be early hair loss, finger nail ridging, with discoloration. Allodynia is noted.
Stage III: Pain is no longer sympathetically maintained. There is atrophy and joint dysfunction.
Stage IV: Final stage is with a useless hand and numerous systemic symptoms: immune system failure, orthostatic hypotension, and severe depression.

TREATMENT

Early recognition and early management is paramount. Multidisciplinary care must be instituted early, as simple, single monotherapy leads to failure. Merely a nerve block, a stellate ganglion block, or nonspecific physical therapy does not suffice. All and more are needed.

Physical Therapy

Active range of motion of all the upper extremity joints "as tolerated by the patient" must be initiated. Pain aggravation by any activity must be avoided, as distress from pain aggravation exacerbates sympathetic dysfunction.

Local ice application in a limited time frame (several seconds) followed by heat applications are effective in the early acute stage to relieve pain and minimize edema. General inactivity must be avoided, as it fosters dependency, depression, and loss of general function.

Treatment of edema is mechanically addressed by compressive dressings. In the fingers and hand, string applied from distal to proximal and repeatedly applied is effective and can be applied by the patient using the normal hand if the mental status is deemed appropriate (Figure 12.8). Edema can also be decreased by magnesium sulphate (Epsom salts) taken orally or rectally by enema.

Pain relief is the top priority. No patient can overcome or prevent loss of function or restore function if pain is not properly controlled. The ideal analgesic is antidepressant medication.[22–24] Antidepressants also create endorphins as well as combat depression.

Psychological factors are considered pertinent in chronic pain, as are psychosocial factors, but their effect on acute pain has not been adequately studied. This involves temporal factors, as acute pain is brief and chronic after a longer duration. Some studies are emphasizing the effects of psychological factors, especially depression, in initiating pain perception and its significance.[25–27]

Drug Therapy

Opiates may play a major role in pain management of CRPS. The opioid agonist buprenorphine neutralizes the unwanted side effects of opioids. Anticonvulsants are also effective in CRPS.[25,26]

Nonsteroidal anti-inflammatory drugs are effective in relieving the inflammatory aspects of CRPS and must be carefully monitored to minimize or avoid gastric side effects. The alpha$_1$-blockers phenoxybenzamine (Dibenzyline) and clonidine administered orally, intrathe-

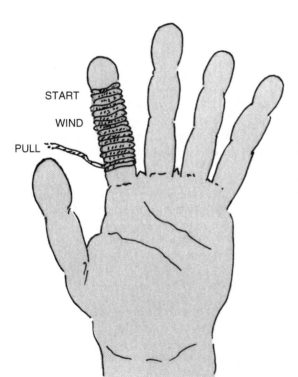

START

WIND

PULL

Figure 12.8 String application for finger edema. A large string wrapped from the distal aspects of the finger and gradually wrapped proximally decreases edema. Once applied, it is removed and reapplied until the edema is gone or significantly diminished. It must be applied several times daily. (Reprinted with permission from Cailliet R. *The Shoulder in Hemiplegia*. Philadelphia: F.A. Davis, 1980;118.)

cally, or by patch are effective if the patch is not applied locally over the hyperpathic area but is applied paravertebrally instead.[28,29] Analgesic somatic nerve blocks, compressive regional blocks, or sympathetic ganglion nerve blocks all belong in the armamentarium of treatment.

Surgical Therapy

Surgical sympathectomy may be considered when local blocks are effective, but there is recurrence or persistence of symptoms. The side effects of these blocks, such as persistent Horner's syndrome, must be carefully evaluated and accepted by the patient and family.

SUMMARY

It is apparent from the multiple modalities indicated above that treatment of CRPS must be multidisciplinary from the start, with the avoidance of merely one form of treatment. All of these possible treatment procedures may not be in the expertise of the primary physician but must be known to exist so that appropriate referral occurs early.

REFERENCES

1. Davis SW, *et al*. Shoulder-hand syndrome in a hemiplegic population: A 5 year retrospective study. *Arch Phys Med Rehabil* 1977;58:353–356.
2. Lusskin R, *et al*. Rehabilitation surgery on adult spastic hemiplegia. *Lin Orthop* 1969;63:32.
3. Coventry MB. Problem of the painful shoulder. *JAMA* 1953;177:153.
4. Moskowitz E, *et al*. Posthemiplegic reflex sympathetic dystrophy. *JAMA* 1958;167:836–838.
5. Cailliet R. *The Shoulder in Hemiplegia*. Philadelphia: F.A. Davis, 1980.
6. Kosin F. Painful Shoulder and the Reflex Sympathetic Dystrophy Syndrome. In: McCarthy DJ (ed). *Arthritis and Allied Conditions: A Textbook of Rheumatology*. Philadelphia: Lea & Febiger, 1979.
7. Merskey H, Bogduk N. *Classification of Chronic Pain Descriptions of Chronic Pain Syndromes and Definitions of Pain Terms, second edition*. Seattle: IASP Press, 1994.
8. Bruehl S, *et al*. External validation of IASP diagnostic criteria for complex regional pain syndrome and proposed research diagnostic criteria. *Pain* 1999;81:147–154.
9. Drummond PD, *et al*. Reflex sympathetic dystrophy: the significance of differing plasma catecholamine concentrations in affected and unaffected limbs. *Brain* 1991;114:2025–2036.
10. Kolzenburg K, McMahon SB. The enigmatic role of the sympathetic nervous system in chronic pain. *Trends Pharmacol Sci* 1991;12:399–402.

11. Sweet WH, Poletti CE. Causalgia and Sympathetic Dystrophy (Sudek's Atrophy). In: Aronoff GM (ed). *Evaluation and Treatment of Chronic Pain*. Baltimore: Urban & Swchwartzenberg, 1985;149–165.

12. Guyton AC. *Basic Neuroscience, second edition*. Philadelphia: W.B. Saunders, 1991.

13. Koltzenberg M. Stability and plasticity of nociceptor function. *IASP Newsletter* 1995;January/February:3–4.

14. Willis WD, Westlund KN. Neuroanatomy of the pain system and the pathways that modulate pain. *J Clin Neurophysiol* 1997;14(1):2–31.

15. Arnold JM, *et al.* Increased venous alpha-adrenoceptor responsiveness in patients with reflex dystrophy. *Ann Intern Med* 1993;118:619–621.

16. Berkley KJ, Hubscher CH. Are there separate central nervous system pathways for touch and pain? *Nat Med* 1985;1:766–773.

17. Benarroch EE. The central autonomic network: Functional organization, dysfunction and perspective. *Mayo Clin Proc* 1993;68:988–1001.

18. Blumberg H, Janig W. Clinical manifestations of reflex sympathetic dystrophy and sympathetically maintained pain. In: Wall PD, Melzack R (eds). *Text Book of Pain*. Edinburgh: Churchill Livingstone, 1994;685–698.

19. Sato J, Perl EB. Adrenogenic excitation of cutaneous pain receptors induced by peripheral nerve injury. *Science* 1991;25:1608–1610.

20. Taber C, *et al.* Measurement of reactive dilation during cold gel pack application of nontraumatized ankles. *Phys Ther* 1992;72:294–299.

21. Low PA, *et al.* Quantitative sudomotor axon reflex in normal and neuropathic subjects. *Ann Neurol* 1983;14:573–580.

22. American Academy of Neurology. Therapeutic and Technology Assessment Subcommittee. Thermography in neurological practice. *Neurology* 1990;40:523–525.

23. Wahren LK, Torebjork HE. Quantitative sensory test in patients with neuralgia 11 to 25 years after injury. *Pain* 1992;48:237–244.

24. Ardid D, Guilbaud G. Antinociceptive effects of acute and "chronic" injections of tricyclic antidepressant drugs in a new model of mono-neuropathy in rats. *Pain* 1992;49:279–287.

25. McQuay H, *et al.* A systematic review of antidepressants in neuropathic pain. *Pain* 1996;68:217–227.

26. Ollat H, Cesaro P. Pharmacology of neuropathic pain. *Clin Neuropharmacol* 1995;18:391–404.

27. Linton SJ. A review of psychological risk factors in back and neck pain. *Spine* 2000;25:1148–1156.

28. Wilton TD. Tegretol in the treatment of diabetic neuropathy. *S Afr Med J* 1974;48:869–872.

29. Rull JA, *et al.* Symptomatic treatment of peripheral diabetic neuropathy with carbamazepine (Tegretol) double blind cross over trial. *Diabetologia* 1969;5:215–218.

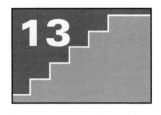

Flexor Synergy of the Upper Extremity after Hemorrhagic Stroke

Rene Cailliet

Restoration of function of the hand, fingers, and wrist after completed stroke must take into consideration the neurologic aspect of the distal portion of the upper extremity. The flexor synergy that occurs as compared to the extensor synergy of the lower extremity has the following components.

The shoulder girdle in the hemiplegic spastic phase has been addressed in Chapter 11. As noted, the elbow flexes, the forearm pronates, the wrist flexes, the fingers flex and adduct, and the thumb flexes in conjunction with internal rotation of the shoulder.

Although the flexor synergy is predominant, occasionally, an extensor synergy of the upper extremity can occur in which the elbow extends with pronation of the forearm, the wrist extends somewhat, the fingers flex with adduction, and the thumb adducts in flexion. It is apparent that in the extensor synergy only the elbow and forearm varies from the flexor synergy.

On analysis, any treatment approach must address activities of daily living. Thus, therapeutic approaches should consider function rather than isolation of individual muscle groups, although the latter, obviously, must be evaluated in examining the difficulties of the patient performing activities of daily living.

Research in animals who have been selectively impaired from cortical ablation have been noted to undergo cortical reorganization. This reorganization originally has been in the sensory sphere, but, more recently, complex reorganization of the motor cortex has been described.[1–3]

In the subacute stage of the completed stroke, there is a decrease in motor cortex excitability and in the size of the cortical representation area of the paretic muscles in the premotor cortex.[4,5] This decrease may be the result of disuse but could be due to damage of the neural structures of the cortex. Constraint-induced (CI) therapy has been shown in controlled studies[1] to improve function and also increase the area of cortical representation in the premotor cortex.

This does not mean that CI therapy is the only or the best manner of providing functional rehabilitation, but it does open an encouraging aspect of therapeutic involvement, with objective measurement of the size of the active cerebral cortex that has been damaged by stroke. As these studies have been conducted months after stroke, they also lend credence to pursuing treatment for longer periods than is frequently undertaken.

CI therapy involves immobilization of the normal contralateral arm and hand while the patient undergoes rehabilitation treatment for the impaired arm. The patients in the Liepert et al. study,[1] which lasted 12 days, were able to extend their wrists 20 degrees and their fingers 10 degrees, and they were able to walk during the period of shoulder and arm immobilization. Excluded from the study were patients with serious medical problems, global aphasia, cognitive impairment that precluded the ability to comply with instructions in motor testing, and epilepsy and those wearing a cardiac pacemaker. The latter was because these patients were being studied with magnetic resonance imaging instruments.

The patients were immobilized comfortably with a shoulder, arm, and hand-finger splint for 9 hours a day. They were released only during sleeping hours. During their immobilization, they underwent several periods of occupational physical therapy in hand-finger activities. The type of therapy was the standard.[6–8]

Rehabilitation modalities of hand function vary regarding "exercise therapy," which aims at restoring individual hand-finger function. Many evolved in treatment for cerebral palsied children but ultimately were applied to adults and stroke patients.

Fay[9] suggested the use of pathologic and unlocking reflexes. The Bobaths[10] also developed a neurodevelopmental treatment program in which they postulated that normal motor performance was inhibited by sensory disturbances, spasticity, disturbances of postural reflex mechanisms, and loss of selective movement patterns. Brunnstrom[11] proposed muscle re-education using reflex training. She defined the associated reactions of hemiplegia as involuntary limb movements revoked by yawning, sneezing, and coughing, and used the labyrinthic and tonic neck reflexes. She also used resistance to the "normal" extremity and tapping and stroking for sensory stimulation.

Knott,[12] quoting Kabat, developed the neuromuscular facilitation system in which the total (synergistic) patterns were invoked and resistance given to the portion of the extremity desired. These techniques included maximum resistance, repetition, traction, and use of verbal commands. Basic spiral diagonal patterns of movement were used.

Rood stressed sensory input to enhance motor response.[13] She stimulated skin receptors by ice application, stroking, and brushing. Basmajian[14] used biofeedback. All of these techniques are described in Chapter 4 of Basmajian's text.[15]

Stern[16] studied the value of facilitation techniques versus a traditional type of exercise program and showed that either or both benefited the patient equally. Basmajian[15] summarized the value of exercise programs as "Most current hemiplegic exercise programs tend to be an eclectic combination of traditional methods, neuromuscular facilitation techniques, biofeedback training and sensorimotor therapy." With magnetic resonance imaging PETY studies, as stated by Liepert et al.,[1] differentiation may evolve that will standardize and equate benefit from one of the current programs.[15]

Immediately after the "completion" of a stroke, there is paralysis or paresis of the upper extremity musculature, with initial weakness noted in the distal musculature, especially the intrinsics of the hand. Gradually, the weakness occurs in the forearm, arm, and then shoulder, in that order. The deep tendon reflexes are lost, and hypotonia occurs.

Sensory dysfunction of pain sensation, proprioception, light touch, and vibration occurs. Two-point discrimination, stereognosis, and graphesthesia are lost, which makes the hand and fingers nonfunctional. If there are perceptual and visual dysfunctions, they also adversely affect the hand. Spontaneous motor recovery occurs chiefly within the initial 2–3 months after the stroke, with the first voluntary movements noted 6–33 days after onset. Recovery at first is that of flexor synergy, which then leads to return of voluntary control of the components or all of the synergy. The intent of therapy is this return from involuntary synergy on stimulus to voluntary control.

Return of meaningful, voluntary control of hand function varies from 20% to 40% of patients having total recovery to the remainder having no functional recovery.[17] Carroll[18] stated in 1986 that if there was no motor functional return in the first week, it was considered unlikely that the patient would regain full use of the involved hand. More recent studies have not refuted this opinion, but from review of plasticity in recent neurophysiologic studies, this pessimistic prognosis may change.

REFERENCES

1. Liepert J, *et al*. Treatment-induced cortical reorganization after stroke in humans. *Stroke* 2000;31:1210–1216.

2. Merzanich NM, *et al.* Somatosensory cortical map changes following digital amputation in adult monkeys. *J Comp Neurol* 1984;224:591–605.

3. Weiller C, *et al.* Functional reorganization of the brain in recovery from striatocapsular infarction in man. *Ann Neurol* 1992;32:463–472.

4. Cacinelli P, *et al.* Post-stroke reorganization of brain motor output to the hand: A 2–4 month followup with focal magnetic transcranial stimulation. *Electromyogr Clin Neurophysiol* 1997;105:438–450.

5. Rossini PM, *et al.* Hand motor cortical area reorganization in stroke: A study with iMRI, MBG, and TCS maps. *Neuroreport* 1998;9:2141–2146.

6. Duncan PW. Synthesis of intervention trials to improve motor recovery following stroke. *Top Stroke Rehabil* 1997;3:1–20.

7. Twitchell TH. The restoration of motor function following hemiplegia in man. *Brain* 1951;74:443–480.

8. Bard O, Hirschberg GG. Recovery of voluntary motor recovery in upper extremity following hemiplegia. *Phys Med Rehabil* 1965;46:567–572.

9. Fay T. The use of pathological and unlocking reflexes in the rehabilitation of spastics. *Am J Phys Med* 1954;33:347–352.

10. Bobath B. Treatment of adult hemiplegia. *Physiotherapy* 1977;63:310–313.

11. Brunnstrom S. *Movement Therapy in Hemiplegia.* New York: Harper & Row, 1970.

12. Knott M, Voss DE. *Proprioceptive Neuromuscular Facilitation.* New York: Harper & Row, 1968.

13. Stockmeyer SA. An interpretation of the approach of Rood to the treatment of neuromuscular dysfunction. *Am J Phys Med* 1967;46:900–956.

14. Basmajian JV. Biofeedback in rehabilitation: A review of principles and practices. *Arch Phys Med Rehabil* 1981;62:469–475.

15. Basmajian JV. *Therapeutic Exercises, fourth edition.* Baltimore: Williams & Wilkins, 1984.

16. Stern PH, et al. Effects of facilitation exercise techniques in stroke rehabilitation. *Arch Phys Med Rehabil* 1970;51:526–531.

17. Lieberman JS. Hemiplegia: Rehabilitation of the Upper Extremity. In: Kaplan PE, Cerullo LJ (eds), *Stroke Rehabilitation.* Boston: Butterworth, 1986;95–117.

18. Carroll D. Hand function in hemiplegia. *J Chron Dis* 1986;18:493–500.

14 Lower Extremity in Stroke

Rene Cailliet

Paralysis of the extremities in acute stroke heralds a bad prognosis. Only one-third of patients who do not die from the hemorrhage and who have paralysis of the lower extremity regain walking function.[1] The Copenhagen Stroke Study indicates that only 10% of stroke patients with leg paralysis achieve walking function.[1] Walking prognosis, therefore, is important, as it also determines the patient's independence.[2,3]

Predicting the prognosis is important to assure the patient and the family of future rehabilitation efforts. Two factors have been of predictive value: the patient's ability to cope with activities of daily living and the development of lower extremity strength during the first week.[3] Age did not influence the prediction of ultimate walking.

The size of the cerebral lesion also did not influence the prognosis, implying that recovery was related to the functional potential of the unaffected, undamaged portion of the cortex and the contralateral side.

There is a perceptual difference between patients with stroke from infarct and from intracerebral hemorrhage, which also influences recovery. Perception can be viewed as a process of interacting with the environment, which includes motor skills, sensory integration, visual perception, cognition, and psychological and social components.[4] The higher-level perceptual functions tend to be relatively susceptible to intracerebral stroke pathology early in the disease, translating to an adverse implication for prognosis of functional recovery.

GAIT RECOVERY AFTER STROKE

Before discussion of the stroke gait can be analyzed, normal gait must be addressed. The initiation of walking from a stance posture results from "the body losing its balance as a result of cessation of activity of the postural muscles which include the erector spinae and certain thigh and leg muscles."[5] The next phase is forward propulsion. As the center of gravity moves forward, the stance foot and leg bear the weight, and the other lower limb moves forward to prevent the entire body from falling.

> The force that produces forward progression in gait is the potential energy obtained as the body falls ahead of the supporting foot (leg). Kinetic energy is gained in this fall and is then used to regain potential energy when the body is lifted up over the contra lateral foot in the next support phase.[6]

Normal gait is symmetric both in time and distance. The left supports the right and vice versa, and the step lengths are equal. Economic walking speed is approximately 120 steps per minute, with increase in velocity occurring by decreasing the stride cadence and increasing the length of the stride. When walking speeds are decreased to fewer than 70 steps per minute, the pelvis no longer rotates and the arms no longer swing in an alternate manner.[7]

Walking is a "rhythmic displacement of bodily parts that maintains the animal in constant forward progression over a level surface. The erect bipedal locomotion is a relatively prolonged affair and appears to be a learned process not the inborn reflexes."[8] As walking is a learned process, each individual displays certain peculiarities, but all are superimposed on a basic pattern of bipedal locomotion.[8]

Walking occurs in cycles, with each cycle being the same as the preceding. A cycle involves both stance and swing. The erect body is supported first on one leg then the other as the other leg "swings" forward in preparation for the next stance phase. One foot is always on the ground, meaning that proper proprioception is needed if the stance phase has any time frame.

At each step, the body speeds up then slows down and rises and falls as the body passes over the stance phase when the supporting leg is erect. The distance of rising is only a few centimeters but, with the body weight, that requires significant energy. Certain aspects of gait, termed *determinants of gait*, help to conserve this energy.

These determinants are lateral shift of the pelvis, rotation of the pelvis, flexion of the knee during the stance phase, and flexion extension of the foot and ankle. This is a complex, integrated phenomenon that is inborn and modified by time and use as well as practice (Figure 14.1). If any component is lost, as in a completed stroke, gait is impaired.

During gait progression, the foot is dorsiflexed at heel strike, but, as this occurs by the anterior tibialis muscle, the foot also supinates. At midstance, the foot is "flat" and pronates, remaining so until the heeloff phase when the foot again supinates as it dorsiflexes (Figure 14.2).

The pelvis during gait has determinants to diminish the elevation and depression of the pelvis as it laterally flexes and rotates. This infers

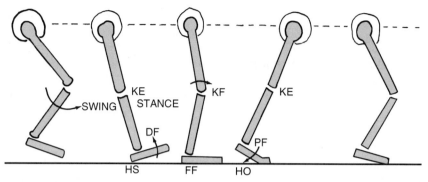

Figure 14.1 Gait components. Viewed laterally, the gait sequence (of one leg). The swing phase goes into the stance phase at heel strike (HS) where the knee is extended (KE). The ankle is dorsiflexed (DF). As the body passes over the center of gravity, the knee flexes slightly (KF) to prevent the hip rising significantly above the horizontal (*dotted line*). Further progression finds knee extension and heel off (HO) and the foot plantar flexed (PF), then there is the beginning of another swing phase. (FF = foot flat.)

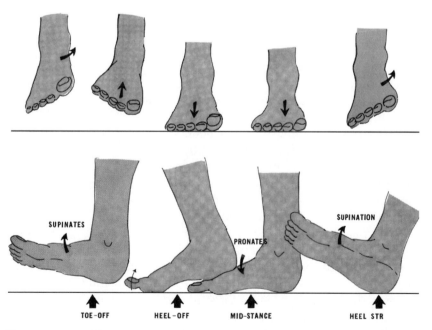

Figure 14.2 The foot during gait. At heel strike (HEEL STR), the foot is supinated as well as dorsiflexed as it has been during the swing phase. At midstance, the foot flattens to the ground and pronates, remaining so until heel-off when supination and dorsiflexion again are regained for the swing phase. (Reprinted with permission from Cailliet R. *Foot and Ankle Pain, third edition.* Philadelphia: F.A. Davis, 1997;64.)

that the erector spinae paraspinous muscles also alternately contract and relax in synchrony with the rest of gait.

It can be noted that many of the muscular activities of the leg, knee, and ankle during gait require flexion patterns. These are lost after a stroke, which releases the extensor patterns.

The hip flexors during the swing phase are replaced by the hip extensor (gluteals) and knee extensors (quadriceps) during the heel strike phase. The hamstring muscles (hip flexors) that decelerate the swinging leg also are lost in the gait pattern.

At midstance, the knee normally flexes slightly to diminish pelvic elevation. The extensor pattern of stroke patients denies this relaxation, and the knee remains extended, making the leg longer, and the patient "compensates" by swinging the leg in abduction to clear the floor.

The gastrocsoleus muscle that plantar flexes the foot normally reciprocally relaxes to permit the anterior tibialis to dorsiflex and supinate the foot. In the stroke extensor synergy, the gastrocsoleus muscle remains contracted, inhibiting ankle dorsiflexion and supination. The expected dorsiflexion of the foot to clear the floor during the swing phase is lost, and the patient cannot clear the floor during swing. Stumbling and even tripping may occur with a fall, as the patient is uncoordinated and has impaired proprioception.

During hemiplegic gait, which is now asymmetric as to time and distance, the normal leg swings faster to minimize the duration of the stance phase on the impaired leg. Due to insecurity, the total gait is slowed; thus, the trunk muscles also are impaired, and the alternate arm swing aspect is lost.

During the swing phase, as has been stated, the ankle must dorsiflex to clear the floor as part of the flexion pattern at the hip and knee. The peronei, which are evertors of the foot, should be relaxed, as the anterior tibialis, supinator, and dorsiflexors are active. Stroke patients lose this balance. Function of the peroneus longus muscle, which helps to stabilize the foot during midstance, is also lost.[10]

As the patient attempts to perform the swing phase of gait with the spastic leg, the swing leg should undergo significant flexion to clear the floor, but, due to hypertonus of the extensor muscles, no flexion can occur. The knee remains extended and the foot in plantar flexion. The only way the leg can be swung forward and clear the floor is by hiking the hip on that side and circumducting the leg during the swing phase.

At the end of the swing phase, when heel strike is normal, the plantar-flexed ankle and foot, the ball of the foot, and the metatarsal heads strike the ground first. The foot often remains outwardly rotated as the pelvis elevates and rotates.

The extensor pattern implies loss of reciprocal relaxation. With the pelvis elevated, the hip flexes in external rotation and abduction, reflexively flexing the knee, and the foot reflexively dorsiflexes and supinates with the toes flexed. This anterior tibialis action persists throughout the forward movement. Another pattern has been implemented.

Most patients who undergo this spastic swing phase have difficulty in transferring their weight over the sound leg, resulting in too much weight being borne by the hemiplegic leg. In attempting to initiate the swing phase, the foot is stimulated by the ground pressure against the spastic foot, and more extensor action occurs with no reciprocal flexion.

The knee is never fully extended during normal gait, with the small degree of flexion (5–10 degrees) acting as a shock absorber and permitting normal determinants. Without a slight flexion during midstance, the other leg cannot appropriately flex.

Because the patient does not normally have control of his or her hip extensor, as the hemiplegic patient steps forward on the normal side, the hemiplegic leg moves backward, interfering with forward translation. This backward motion of the hemiplegic leg causes the knee to hyperextend, being limited only by the soft tissues—the ligaments and the capsules—which can cause pain.

TREATMENT

The therapist, after analyzing the faulty gait pattern, applies her or his hands to assist the desired pattern and prevent the unwanted aspects of the spastic pattern.[11] Balance, stance, and weight transfer must be practiced.

Preparation for standing from sitting must be initiated and practiced before walking is attempted. Immediately on gaining weightbearing, the hemiplegic limb "prematurely" contracts into total extensor pattern from weightbearing stimulation of the foot against the ground, causing the leg to extend before the body passes over the center of gravity.[12] The therapist manually assists the patient to stand then walk to facilitate more normal patterns and minimize unwanted patterns, which means weight balance by transfer over the center of gravity.

The Bobath technique attempts recovery by manually assisting the patient to regain normal active functional patterns. This differs for exercising individual muscles, albeit their being in the attempted patterns, or even exercising the muscles in total but non–weightbearing patterns.[13]

Therapy attempts to restore normal function to the degree of restoration of the activities of daily living. How and which therapy achieves this remain unanswered questions, but some developments outlined in the following sections are encouraging. Numerous other treatment procedures are well illustrated in the literature and are not duplicated in this text.[14]

Constraint-Induced Movement Therapy

Involving the "plasticity" of the central nervous system, constraint-induced movement therapy is an exciting therapeutic intervention that has been postulated by the University of Alabama and the Freidrich Schiller University of Jena Germany. This approach has been essentially used in the upper extremity but is contemplated for the lower extremity. Under this approach, the unaffected side is immobilized so that the patient must attempt to use the impaired extremity for normal, familiar daily tasks. Through constraint-induced movement therapy, the portion of the brain that normally performs these functions doubles in size.[15] The immobilization of the unaffected side must be applied 6 hours a day for 90% of waking hours and applied for at least 2 weeks, during which the patient performs physical and occupational therapy for the non-immobilized (hemiplegic) arm. After a stroke, many cells die and many that remain are nonfunctional. It is these nonfunctional cells that apparently are "stimulated" to make synaptic connection through constraint-induced movement therapy.

Bracing

Bracing to minimize plantar flexion of the foot has been universally used. There are numerous types of braces, but their function is to dorsiflex the foot as much as possible and minimize plantar flexion. A form-fitting plastic brace molded to the patient's leg, ankle, and foot, with the foot as close to 90 degrees of flexion as possible, is currently the most popular and effective.

Medications for Spasticity

There are numerous medications used to diminish spasticity, including Baclofen (Lioresal). This is a gamma-aminobutyric acid (GABA) that decreases monosynaptic and polysynaptic transmission in the spinal cord. Spasticity is allegedly decreased, as GABA prevents uptake of calcium, which is required for the release of excitatory neurotransmitters such as glutamate and aspartate. Baclofen is absorbed quickly from the gastrointestinal tract but crosses the blood barrier poorly. Baclofen is started at 5–10 mg per day, gradually increasing to 40 mg per day.

Diazepam (Valium) is a benzodiazepine derivative that has a direct effect as a GABA receptor agonist and allows flow of calcium across the nerve membrane. Diazepam has undesirable side effects, including sedation, weakness, and depression. It is administered in 2-mg tablets starting with divided doses two to three times a day as tolerated.

Dantrolene sodium (Dantrium) does not act on the central nervous system but has direct effect on skeletal muscle. It inhibits the release of calcium from the cytoplasmic reticulum into the sarcoplasm of skeletal muscles. It is hepatotoxic in addition to causing generalized weakness and lethargy. Begun at 25 mg daily, it is gradually increased to 400 mg daily in divided doses.

Clonazepam (Klonopin) is also a benzodiazepine derivative that is primarily used for epilepsy but has been noted to decrease spasticity. In 0.5-mg tablets, the initial dose is one tablet at bedtime with gradual increase as tolerated.

Neuromuscular block injections into the muscles at their myoneural junctions have also been used. The muscle considered to cause the major impairment is chosen. There are three commonly used medications: 45% ethyl alcohol in sterile saline, phenol in 4–6% aqueous solution, and botulinum toxin. Use of 45% ethyl alcohol has undergone no placebo-controlled double-blind studies, and it can cause local muscle damage, so it is infrequently used.

Phenol (4–6% aqueous solution) is injected into motor points of selected muscles under electromyogram guidance or into a surgically exposed nerve to assure that the nerve is strictly motor and not sensory. If injected in the vicinity of a sensory nerve, a severe pain can result. Injection into a motor nerve causes wallerian degeneration, with ultimate regeneration, and the effect can last 3–18 months. This injection must be performed in a hospital setting, as general anesthesia is needed, and it is time consuming, as precise electromyographic localization of the motor nerve is required.

Botulinum toxin type A (Botox) has also been used in hypertonia from stroke. It is a neurotoxin that blocks the neuromuscular junction, but the injection does not require motor point localization; instead, merely finding the target muscle is sufficient.[16] No general anesthesia is needed. Twelve to 24 hours are needed before its effect is noted, and the effect can last 36 months before reinjection can be given. The dose is 4–10 U/kg of body weight (300–400 U at one time). Botulinum can also be used when a mild contracture occurs that requires casting. Its effect is recoverable.

PAIN IN THE HEMIPLEGIC PATIENT

Pain from faulty biomechanics of the foot, ankle, and knee due to stroke must be minimized, as pain deters patient function as well as adding depression when it persists. Shoulder pain was discussed in Chapter 11.

The foot, which normally bears weight at the posterior heel (calcaneus) on heel strike, does not undergo this mechanism after stroke, as the foot is plantar flexed and the heel does not strike. The foot is supinated and plantar flexed during swing phase and enters heel strike at the midstance phase (Figure 14.3).

The supinated plantar flexed foot places the peroneal tendon and muscle under stress, and tendonitis of the peroneus may occur. Clinically, this tendon can be identified by the patient and tenderness elicited by manually pressing on it. Bracing to minimize supination, oral anti-inflammatory medications, and local ice then heat are effective pain control measures. If pain is severe and persistent, a local injection of an analgesic and steroid into the sheath is effective.

As the foot becomes weightbearing in midstance, the foot pronates and the metatarsal head becomes weightbearing, often with impact from the irregular gait pattern. Pain is felt over the metatarsal head on the plantar surface. The pain is located by manually pressing over the metatarsal head, which elicits the identical pain. In weightbearing, the foot is also seen as being pronated and all the metatarsal heads equally on the ground.

Treatment is to minimize or avoid contact of the second, third, and even fourth metatarsal heads with the ground. This is done by placing a metatarsal pad behind the metatarsal heads and even incorporating this pad into the plastic lower extremity brace.

"Back knee" when the leg becomes weightbearing occurs because the plantar flexed ankle cannot sufficiently dorsiflex, and, hence, the leg goes into hyperextension at the knee. This may be corrected

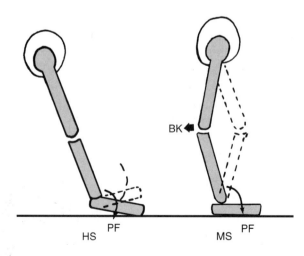

Figure 14.3
Mechanisms of back knee (BK) in hemiplegia. Heel strike (HS) is shown on the left. The plantar flexed foot (PF) strikes the toes rather than the heel. At midstance (MS), the plantar flexed foot causes the knee to hyperextend (BK).

by ankle-foot bracing, but, if not, a knee bra
hyperextension.

CONCLUSION

As stated, only a small percentage of patients who have had a
especially a hemorrhagic stroke, regain satisfactory functional an
lation. The Copenhagen Stroke Study Group has developed a prelih
inary index for estimating the prognosis of regaining satisfactory gait.
For those patients who undergo rehabilitation, techniques for recovery have been postulated, and, with further studies, better results will
be possible. Independence is the aim of rehabilitation, and regaining a
safe gait is needed for independent living.

REFERENCES

1. Jorgensen HS, *et al.* Recovery of walking function in stroke: The Copenhagen Stroke Study. *Arch Phys Med Rehabil* 1995;76:27–35.
2. Bohannon RW, *et al.* Importance of four variables of walking to patients with stroke. *Int J Rehabil Res* 1991;14:246–250.
3. Wandel A, *et al.* Prediction of walking function in stroke patients with initial lower extremity paralysis: The Copenhagen Stroke Study. *Arch Phys Med Rehabil* 2000;81:736–738.
4. Su C-Y, *et al.* Perceptual differences between stroke patients with cerebral infarction and intracerebral hemorrhage. *Arch Phys Med Rehabil* 2000;81:706–714.
5. Carloo S. The initiation of walking. *Acta Anat* 1966;65:1–9.
6. Klein-Vogelbach S. *Funktionelle Bewegungslehre Rehabilitation und Pravention, volume 1.* New York: Springer, Berlin Heidelberg, 1976.
7. Wall JC, Ashburn A. Assessment of gait disability in hemiplegics. Hemiplegic gait. *Scand J Rehabil Med* 1979;11:95–103.
8. Inman VT, *et al. Human Walking.* Baltimore: William & Wilkins, 1981.
9. Saunders JB, *et al.* The major determinants in normal and pathological gait. *J Bone Joint Surg* 1953;35A:543.
10. Walmsley RP. Electromyographic study of the phasic activity of peroneus longus and brevis. *Arch Phys Med Rehabil* 1977;58:6–69.
11. Bobath B (ed). *Adult Hemiplegia: Evaluation and Treatment.* London: Heinemann, 1978.
12. Knuttson E. Gait control in hemiparesis. *Scand J Rehabil Med* 1981;13:101–108.
13. Voss DI. What's the answer? *Phys Ther* 1969;49:1030.
14. Davies PM. *Steps to Follow: A Guide to the Treatment of Adult Hemiplegia.* New York: Springer-Verlag, 1985.
15. Liepert J, *et al.* Treatment-induced cortical reorganization after stroke in humans. *Stroke* 2000;31:1210–1216.
16. Brin M (ed). Spasticity: Etiology, evaluation, management and role of botulinum toxin A. *Muscle Nerve* 1997;Suppl 6:S1–S232.

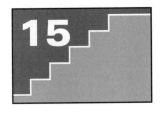

15 Musculoskeletal Painful Conditions Resulting from Hemorrhagic Stroke

Rene Cailliet

The most prevalent musculoskeletal pain resulting from the hemorrhagic stroke is the painful shoulder, which has been extensively discussed in Chapters 12 and 13. This has been discussed as the flail shoulder with subluxation in the initial flail arm. Later, in the spastic shoulder, the usual conditions of the rotator cuff can also occur.

The tendonitis of the supraspinatus tendon is prevalent, as the external rotation needed to externally rotate the arm during overhead elevation is lost in the stroke patient due to the spasticity of the subscapularis muscle overwhelming the external rotators: the supraspinatus, infraspinatus, and teres minor muscles. The combined tendon of the rotator cuff impinges on the overhead acromium and the coracoacromial ligament.[1,2]

Clinically, this is apparent, as there is local pain when the arm reaches approximately 90 degrees of abduction. When this has occurred many times, the rotator cuff may be frayed and even torn. If the tear is partial, the clinical picture is the same as that of tendonitis, with the torn collagen fibers of the cuff bunching up and sufficient fibers remaining intact to abduct and flex the arm.

If the rotator cuff is totally torn, there is no longer the ability to initiate abduction and forward flexion of the arm to the degree that invokes deltoid action. The arm also cannot be externally rotated nor sustained in passively incurred horizontal abduction.

Treatment invokes intra-articular injections of a steroid and analgesic agent, oral nonsteroidal anti-inflammatory drugs, and active passive physical therapy, dependent on the stage and degree of the injury.

At the elbow, because the extensors of the wrist and hand originate at the lateral epicondyle, epicondylitis may occur. This is inflammation of the origin of the extensor muscles. There is local tenderness, and pain is accentuated by wrist-finger extension. Treatment is from local injection of an anesthetic agent with steroid into the area.

The wrist presents a major problem, as the hand and fingers are placed into a constant flexed posture due to flexor spasticity. This is the position where hand circulation is minimized, and the hand-finger-shoulder syndrome occurs. This evolution, diagnosis, and treatment have been discussed in Chapters 12 and 13.

At the wrist, because of limited motion and a persistent flexed position, the median nerve at the carpal tunnel can be encroached and inflamed, leading to median nerve compression. In this condition, there is numbness, some pain, and motor loss of the median nerve, involving the thumb and first two fingers.[3] Clinical diagnosis is the reproduction of the symptoms by percussion at the wrist of the median nerve (Tinel sign) and by forceful flexion of the hand. Motor loss is ascertained by weakness of the muscles innervated by the median nerve. Treatment is by a wrist cock-up splint worn daily and at night for several weeks and surgical release if symptoms persist and progress.

The hip presents problems, with a high incidence of fracture from falls due to a precarious balance.[4,5] A hip protector (a modeled pad) that covers the lateral and front side of the hip joint has proven to diminish the incidence of hip fractures and is certainly indicated in stroke patients with a precarious gait.

One of the painful impairments of the knee in the hemiplegic patient is "back knee" (hyperextension) caused by the spasticity of the gastrocsoleus muscle, causing the foot to revert posteriorly (Figures 15.1 and 15.2).[6]

The foot also being malpositioned in the hemiplegic gait presents problems. The foot in normal gait presents heel strike with the foot dorsiflexed and supinated. In hemiplegia, the toes present first, possibly causing metatarsal inflammation. This leads to a condition termed *metatarsalgia*.[7]

Metatarsalgia occurs at the metatarsal heads of the second, third, and fourth metatarsal bone. A properly placed metatarsal pad under the shafts of these three metatarsal bones just proximal to their heads minimizes direct trauma.

As the foot is more supinated than normally, the peroneal muscle and its tendon are placed under stress and become inflamed. This is clinically noted by tenderness over the peroneus tendon. Relief is obtained by a molded arch support, diminishing the degree of supination, and a local injection of an anesthetic agent and steroid into the tendon sheath.

Undoubtedly, other musculoskeletal painful conditions occur in patients with hemorrhagic stroke. The neurologic condition of the stroke invokes a significant alteration of normal musculoskeletal func-

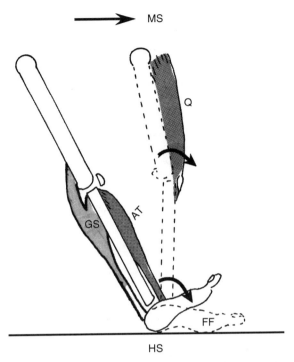

Figure 15.1 Normal gait knee mechanics. At the termination of the swing phase until heel strike (HS), the ankle is dorsiflexed due to contraction of the anterior tibialis (AT) and a relaxed gastrocsoleus (GS) muscle. At midstance (MS), the knee is slightly flexed and the foot "flat" (FF). The quadriceps muscle (Q) allows slight flexion and remains contracted. (Reprinted with permission from Cailliet R. *Foot and Ankle Pain, third edition*. Philadelphia: F.A. Davis, 1997;56.)

tions and thus exposes all of the involved joints to many painful, disabling conditions. Recognition of these conditions leads to a proper diagnosis and therapeutic intervention, but, because of impaired neurologic function, the treatment may be more difficult than in a well person.

Treatment of these and many other conditions requires understanding normal functional anatomy, the tissue site of the pain, and impairment. The therapist is challenged to help the stroke patient overcome impaired neurologic function, which may be difficult to remedy, while at the same time the patient may experience additional pain during therapy, which also impairs desired function and must be addressed.

Approximately 70–80% of patients with stroke have shoulder pain, which includes subluxation, adhesive capsulitis (frozen shoulder), impingement syndrome, rotator cuff tear, brachial plexus traction neuropathies, reflex sympathetic dystrophy, hand-shoulder syndrome,

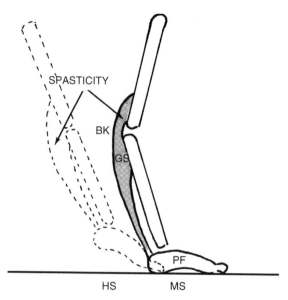

Figure 15.2 Foot and knee mechanics in the hemiplegic patient. Due to spasticity of the gastrocsoleus (GS) muscle, the foot is plantar flexed (PF). There is therefore no heel strike (HS), as the toe touches first. At midstance phase (MS), the foot pronates on the floor but, due to spasticity of the GS muscle to the tibia, is pulled backward, causing a back knee (BK) (hyperextension) at each step.

bursitis, and tendonitis, which have all been mentioned in Chapters 12 and 13. These must be recognized by a careful history and meaningful physical examination, and treatment is dependent on the mechanical findings of the condition.

There also occurs in approximately 5% of patients a central post-stroke pain syndrome that was previously known as *thalamic pain* or *Dejerine-Roussy syndrome*. The common symptoms are pain described as burning and tingling, sharp, stabbing, gnawing, or even dull and achy. These patients exhibit allodynia or hyperpathia, which indicates exaggerated reaction to an otherwise minor stimulus.

Treatment of post-stroke pain syndrome includes general stroke care, such as range-of-motion mobility exercises, imagery, biofeedback, and hypnosis, if they are amenable to the patient's mental status. Medications include analgesics, antidepressants, and anticonvulsants. Neurologic (sympathetic) blocks may be valuable, as is electrical stimulation to the cord. This painful syndrome can tax the expertise of the therapist, as no two patients benefit in the same way from treatment. Depression exists in 10–70% of patients, which enhances or aggravates any pain syndrome and thus must be addressed.

REFERENCES

1. Cailliet R. *Shoulder Pain, third edition.* Philadelphia: F.A. Davis, 1991.
2. Cailliet R. *Soft Tissue Pain and Disability, third edition.* Philadelphia: F.A. Davis, 1996.
3. Cailliet R. *Hand Pain and Impairment, fourth edition.* Philadelphia: F.A. Davis, 1994.
4. Kannus P, *et al.* Prevention of hip fracture in elderly people with use of a hip protector. *N Engl J Med* 2000;343:1506–1512.
5. Hip protectors—A Breakthrough in fracture prevention (editorial). *N Engl J Med* 2000;343:1562–1563.
6. Cailliet R. *Knee Pain and Impairment, third edition.* Philadelphia: F.A. Davis, 1992.
7. Cailliet R. *Foot and Ankle Pain, third edition.* Philadelphia: F.A. Davis, 1997.

Patient with a Hidden Disability

Paul E. Kaplan

Any milieu that reduces patients' abilities to become self-sufficient in their home communities also makes them subject to the prescription and intake of inappropriate medication. Although this situation has not been studied in the stroke population, it has been studied in populations of elderly patients.[1–5] Studies have found that elderly persons have taken inappropriate medications while they were inpatients, outpatients, in extra-care facilities, and in retirement facilities.[6–10] Despite having lists of medications the elderly should avoid, education programs, training projects, and follow-up, errors persist in omission and commission. One of the causative difficulties could be that elderly patients are not necessarily recognized as individuals. If that is a contributing factor, what about the case of the patient with a hidden disability?[11–26] These patients have returned to their home communities but have still not been able to become fully self-sufficient.

HIDDEN DISABILITY SYNDROME

Hidden disability syndrome is an old obstacle faced in rehabilitation medicine.[11,12] It has contributed greatly to the general disability of both chronic pain syndrome and to traumatic brain injury. It produces ineffective, disabled, dependent people. Characteristics of hidden disability syndrome are[12–16]

1. When walking down the street in normal traffic, these patients appear entirely well.
2. These patients have been arbitrarily, unexpectedly subjected to a significant trauma or disease process.
3. The disease process or trauma has significantly disrupted that patient's regular routine, job, daily life, and might have even led to inpatient stays or operative procedures.

4. Although the patient appears healthy, he or she is in fact incapacitated by any number of unseen signs and symptoms, including but not limited to pain, emotional lability, cognitive dysfunction, weakness, sensory deficits, and loss of fine motor coordination.
5. These patients have major issues encompassing anger, dependence, grief, loss, and survivor's guilt.
6. Generally, communities do not highly regard these patients, and they are not well thought of as prime patients for treatment in any practice.

In fact, different medical conditions that contribute to any individual patient's disability can also generate this syndrome. It is prevalent in treating patients with sports injuries, industrial injuries, multiple sclerosis, many of the moderate-to-marked arthritis chronic pain syndromes, psychoses, and cancer.[15–20] It is also prevalent in patients who have had hemorrhagic stroke syndromes.

Generally, hidden disability syndrome is especially observed toward the last stages of the rehabilitative treatment process. Its strategic placement at that position means that how hidden disability syndrome is treated has a large effect on whether that patient will become safely self-sufficient and be able to return to and be accepted to live as a member of his or her home community. Without that acceptance, these patients are often left without friends, family, or future.

PRINCIPLES OF TREATMENT[15–26]

The first principle of treatment is the acquisition of knowledge. The extent of the patient's cognitive deficiency should be determined. Referral to a neuropsychologist for evaluation is extremely important. Even if the patient appears to behave relatively appropriately, neuropsychological examination can delineate cognitive dysfunction. Cognitive dysfunction is frequently accompanied by a reduction in judgment and discrimination. That loss of judgment and discrimination, in turn, ultimately makes the patient less safe and reliable. The patient's self-esteem and self-confidence are greatly reduced. Should the patient have deficits in short-term memory or other cognitive deficiencies, psychological therapy can be applied.

The second principle has to do with the treatment of emotional lability. Rehabilitation psychological support is important at this stage. The therapy—even if begun as an inpatient—is continued during outpatient treatment. Psychological therapy, in these cases, is as important as any advance made in physical therapy or occupational therapy. Quality time should be reserved during the treatment day.

The third principle has to do with team coordination. The psychologist should have a prime role in the coordination or the rehabilitation team's response. That response should be knowledgeable, unified, and harmonious. The effective rehabilitation team is supportive but also supports and maintains external limits to the patient's behavior.

Of the many therapy goals to be achieved, work with the patient's fine motor coordination is strategic. Without that coordination, hundreds of daily tasks become future centers of anxiety and frustration. Even if the patient is relatively bright, it helps if that same patient is also clever enough to create substitutes for many tasks. The therapy itself is not inspiring. It consists of endless repetition, with and without weights. Forming even a simple sequence of new motor actions can require millions of repetitions. Many health clubs provide access to digitally controlled machinery that can generate automatic companionship during that repetition. However, success in these activities is not well represented in national functional outcome monitoring systems.

Access to a safe, heated pool with knowledgeable therapists is beneficial. The heated water reduces muscular spasm and pain. The water reduces strain across major muscles and ligaments. Later, the water provides a medium for resistive and conditioning exercises. Preferred provider system regulations have, however, reduced funding for these types of activities.

SETTING FOR THERAPY

If the patient is agitated, the stakes for successful rehabilitation rise. The patient might at the start of therapy become a part of a dangerous situation. However, many psychiatric facilities are not eager to admit disabled patients. In those that do, the duration of inpatient stays has been shortened. Outpatient therapy is a gamble in that close follow-up is rarely comfortable or convenient. In rural America, outpatient settings could be the only realistic choices.

There are some half-way facilities available for these particular patients. These facilities are often close to larger cities. In these facilities, psychiatry, physical therapy, occupational therapy, recreational therapy, and social work personnel are present or are on call. Nonetheless, preferred provider system financial regulations have reduced financial support for these facilities. Catastrophic insurance programs do not really substitute in these matters. Another obstacle is individual civil rights. Obtaining informed consent might not be easy as well.

FAMILY SUPPORT

The patient's inner circle of friends and family need to support the patient through this difficult time. Nevertheless, that support should be accompanied by support of the rehabilitation team's perceived external limits for the patient's behavior. Communication between that circle of family, friends, and the rehabilitation team should be optimal. That goal is hard to achieve and maintain. Both sides will commonly draw on reserves of goodwill, tolerance of differences in culture, and benevolence of views of the community. During the therapeutic process, these reserves will need to be increased. Counseling can be of great assistance.

MEDICATION

During the treatment period, medications should be minimal yet strong enough to be able to accomplish set objectives. A balance is required. Additionally, the patient will probably take what medications are prescribed for prolonged periods. Medication should be chosen that has few side effects, that is effective for its special task, and that is not expensive or difficult to obtain. Nonsteroidal anti-inflammatory drug therapy for arthritis is a good example, as is medical therapy for diabetes, coronary artery disease, hypertension, and emphysema. Psychotropic medication represents a separate topic, but it should be part of a full psychiatric and psychological follow-up. Using opiate medication is controversial. Enough pain control medication should be given so that the patient is not obstructed in resuming his or her lifestyle. Excessive medication generating patient dependency is a real consideration as well. The balance is realized on a case-by-case basis. The patient should be observed often enough so that an impression is formed of his or her response to pain (pain behavior). Any time patient goals can be realized through non-medicine means, those methods should be preferred.

SPORTS THERAPY

Sports therapy for disabled people has saved and restored many lives. With people who have hidden disabilities, the role of heavily competitive, contact sports is controversial. Many sports, however, are still appropriate, including swimming, walking, hiking, bike riding, boating, and diving. For those patients cognitively challenged, walking or swimming can be closely supervised. Many health clubs provide a variety of conditioning programs at different levels as well as some supervision. Team sports do have their place. Macho-type people often did not do well in the past with hidden disability syndrome after discharge from inpatient rehabilitation. Team sports, such as basketball, touch football, and soccer, have provided an accepted platform for expressing these impulses. Negative impulses have been channeled into team morale activities. Sports therapy clubs and special olympian-type activities have provided an even more demanding venue. Patients who would have been marginal in their response to rehabilitation become enthusiastic, and they are rewarded by feelings of accomplishment.

REFERENCES

1. Zhan C, *et al*. Potentially inappropriate medication use in the community-dwelling elderly. *JAMA* 2001;286:2823.
2. Lindley C, *et al*. Inappropriate medication is a major cause of adverse drug reactions in elderly patients. *Age Ageing* 1992;21:294–300.
3. Gurwitz J, *et al*. Suboptimal medication use in the elderly. *JAMA* 1994;272:316–317.
4. Institute of Medicine. *To Err Is Human*. Washington, DC: National Academy Press, 1999.
5. Nash D, *et al*. *Why the Elderly Need Individualized Pharmaceutical Care*. Philadelphia: Thomas Jefferson University, 2000.
6. Gosney M, Tallis R. Prescription of contraindicated and interacting drugs in elderly patients admitted to the hospital. *Lancet* 1984;2:564–567.
7. Aparasu R, Sitzman S. Inappropriate prescribing for elderly outpatients. *Am J Health Syst Pharm* 1999;56:433–439.
8. Beers MH, *et al*. Inappropriate medicine prescribing in skilled-nursing facilities. *Ann Intern Med* 1992;117:684–689.
9. Golden A, *et al*. Inappropriate medication prescribing in homebound older adults. *J Am Geriatr Soc* 1999;47:948–953.
10. Spore D, *et al*. Inappropriate drug prescriptions for elderly residents of board and care facilities. *Am J Public Health* 1997;87:404–409.
11. American Medical Association. *Handbook of Physical Medicine and Rehabilitation, first edition*. Philadelphia: Blackstone, 1950;484–498.
12. Rusk HA. *Rehabilitation Medicine*. St. Louis: Mosby, 1958;220–232.
13. Critchley M. *The Parietal Lobes*. London: Edward Arnold, 1953;382–386.
14. Goodgold J. *Rehabilitation Medicine*. St. Louis: Mosby, 1988;895–899.
15. Levin HS, *et al*. *Mild Head Injury*. London: Oxford University Press, 1989;247–252.
16. McAlpine D, *et al*. *Multiple Sclerosis*. London: Churchill Livingstone, 1972;216–223.
17. Huelskamp S. Breakthroughs in stroke rehab. *ADVANCE Med Dir Rehab* 2000;9:33–47.
18. Von Korff M, *et al*. Back pain in primary care. Outcomes at 1 year. *Spine* 1993;18:855–862.

19. Von Korff M. Studying the natural history of back pain. *Spine* 1994;19 (18 Suppl):2041S–2046S.
20. Hutter BO, Gilsbach JM. Which neuropsychological deficits are hidden behind a good outcome (Glasgow = 1) after aneurysmal subarachnoid hemorrhage? *Neurosurgery* 1993;33:999–1006.
21. Gordon WA, *et al.* The enigma of "hidden" traumatic brain injury. *J Head Trauma Rehabil* 1998;13:39–56.
22. Rae-Grant AD, *et al.* Sensory symptoms of multiple sclerosis: A hidden reservoir of morbidity. *Mult Scler* 1999;5:179–183.
23. March LM, Brooks PM. Arthritis: The hidden disability. *Med J Aust* 1993;158:369–371.
24. Wagner FA, *et al.* Depression in late life: A hidden public health problem for Mexico? *Salud Publica Mex* 1999;41:189–202.
25. Connolly MJ. Obstructive airways disease: A hidden disability in the aged. *Age Ageing* 1996;25:265–267.
26. Lurie JD, *et al.* A pain in the back. *N Engl J Med* 2000;343:723–726.

Index

Note: Page numbers followed by *f* indicate figures; numbers followed by *t* indicate tables.